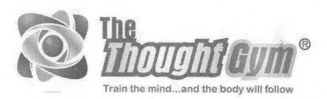

Train the mind...and the body will follow

Hari Kalymnios

www.thethoughtgym.com

The Thought Gym®
First Published 2013

The information contained herein cannot replace or substitute for the services of trained professionals in any field, including but not limited to health or fitness matters. Under no circumstances will Hari Kalymnios or The Thought Gym Ltd or any of its representatives or contractors be liable for any special or consequential damages that result from the use of, or the inability to use, the information or strategies communicated through these materials or any service provided prior to or following the receipt of this book. You alone are responsible and accountable for your decisions, actions and results and by using these materials, you agree not to attempt to hold us liable for any such decisions, actions or results, at any time, under any circumstances.

Every effort has been taken to ensure that we accurately represent these strategies and their potential to help you achieve your health and fitness ambitions. However, we do not purport this as a "quick-fix solution" and there is no guarantee that you will experience any change using the techniques in this program or these materials. Your level of success in attaining results is dependent on a number of factors including (but not limited to) your skill, knowledge, ability, dedication, personality, motivation, focus. Because these (and other) factors vary greatly between individuals we cannot state that you will receive any results as a result of following these materials. These statements and the strategies offered in these materials are simply the author's opinion or experience.

ISBN-13: 978-1481966290

ISBN-10: 1481966294

"The power of the mind – initially sceptical I decided to try it out for myself and give up sugar. Hari was attentive, thorough and very professional in his approach, 10 minutes later and the results speak for themselves – I'm sugar free and proof that the power of the mind really does work!"

Dr Minal Jayakumar, NHS GP

"I saw Hari one time and although I wasn't really planning it, I thought why not and I decided to ask about giving up chocolate. A few weeks later, I forgot about the session and went to a TV commercial casting where I had to pretend that I enjoyed chocolate – I was nearly sick in the studio! I didn't get the job, you may have guessed!"

Brigitte Suligoi, www.basemodels.co.uk

"I am happy to recommend Hari Kalymnios as a professional and talented coach and practitioner. I believe Hari's attention for detail helps him achieve great results with and for those that he works with."

Kate McCartney, www.tobyandkatemccartney.com/

"Hari is a great strategist, thinker & knowledgeable. He is very professional & his attention to detail is unique. I would recommend his services to anyone looking to achieve great results."

Javez Khan, www.javezkhan.com/

"Hari is a very determined, focused and thorough individual. As a client, you can be assured that he won't leave any stone unturned to help you achieve the results and change you are seeking."

J Binning

I dedicate this book to all who wish to regain control over their health and who acknowledge that we are all each personally responsible for our own health and that we have the power to change it.

I look forward to the day when the wave of preventable illnesses, diseases, ailments, aches, pains and obesity incidents fall by the wayside. The first step to achieving this is for people to take personal responsibility for their health, weight, happiness and all other aspects of their lives.

I hope that the ideas, tools and stories in this book inspire you to create positive changes in your life to enable you to live the life that you so richly deserve.

"You don't have to be great to start, but you have to start to be great" – Zig Ziglar

Acknowledgements

I'd like to extend a big "Thank You!" to a few people who helped me with this book.

Huge thanks to my girlfriend and biggest fan, Celest Pereira, for tirelessly reviewing this book on many occasions. I greatly appreciate all the love, support and encouragement that you give me.

Thanks also to my best friend and collaborator in many adventures, Dr Prakash Jayakumar, who reviewed an early draft of this book and made perhaps the most comprehensive annotations ever. I remember our marathon review session vividly.

Thanks to the many other people who took time out of their busy lives to review this book including Alex Kalymnios, Triada Kalymnios, Vijay Kumar, Gemma Clarke, Susanna Pereira, Greg Lowe and Anita Jasser. And thanks to Trevor Uff for helping me to get the cover just right.

And lastly, many thanks and much love to my parents, Dr Demetri and Maria Kalymnios, for - in addition to reviewing and providing feedback on this book - raising me, supporting me and being the best parents that I could wish for.

Contents

9- Exercise

In order to make something of your body, you're going to have to move your body. Understand why it's so important and discover some easy to implement strategies that will help burn those calories effortlessly.

10- Identity & Visualisation

Learn why what you think of yourself is so important for healthy living but also how you can change and improve your identity to fit in with your goals.

11- Goals

Put all you have learnt into practice and follow this method to goal setting to give you the best possible chance of success.

12- A Final Word

Take all you have learnt and get the results you deserve. Keep in touch and remember that if you "train the mind...the body will follow™".

Guided support for the processes in this book can be found using the QR Code below.

1 – Introduction

"Everyone thinks of changing the world, but no one thinks of changing himself" – Leo Tolstoy

"Let him who would move the world, first move himself" - Socrates

This book is designed for anyone who is conscious about their health. Perhaps you recognise that you're mildly overweight or not in as good a shape as you used to be or *can be* – maybe you're totally unfit? Possibly you're overweight or even obese? Whichever it is, if you're not 100% happy with some aspect of your physical being then there will be information in this book that will be of benefit to you and help you to achieve your goals. Even if you think that you're doing well but just want to take better control of your actions with regards to health and fitness, you will get enormous value from this book. I promise you that. My philosophy is that if you 'train the mind...the body will follow™' and it's my aspiration that by reading this book, you will also come to believe this philosophy and make great strides in improving your life.

The chances are that you picked up this book because you (or someone close to you) believed that you have something to gain from what it has to say. Whatever the reasons, whatever the motivation – you're not alone. By picking up and reading this book, you have taken the first step towards an improved 'you'. If you agree, let me guide you over the course of this book on a journey of discovery and realisation that will help you achieve your goals.

I wrote this book because I believe that I can help you. Like many people, I've had my fair share of challenges with living a healthy and fit lifestyle – particularly growing up in a huge city. That's especially true when it comes to eating well and exercising consistently. I'm Greek, and boy, do we know how to eat. As a child and young adult, my eyes really were bigger than my stomach. Exercising - although it was an effort - I worked at it. It was food that was my main weakness. It was always so tasty and plentiful in our family. If there were six of us sitting down for dinner, my Dad would cook for twelve. And I would take it as a personal challenge to fulfil the obligations of the other six!

And it wasn't just eating a lot that was an issue. I didn't have a particularly varied diet growing up. I was a really fussy eater. I used to boast that any exercise I did was for the purposes of 'damage limitation' (i.e. exercise was just to keep at bay all the bad things I was doing to my body elsewhere in my life) and I believed that what I ate didn't matter.

Although I appeared fit (by most people's standards), I wasn't necessarily healthy. In fact, I remember that on my 11th birthday I received a card from one of my sisters with a badge which read *"I built this body on junk food!"* Thinking back, it's funny but I can remember that moment quite vividly. I remember exactly where I was when I first read that. It must have made an impression on me because I often think back to it when I am considering what to eat now.

The thing is though, that even with that jolt at 11, I still didn't make many changes. Hell, I didn't start eating salad until I was 16! Even when I used to go to McDonalds and I used to order the 'HK special' which consisted of 6 chicken McNuggets with bbq sauce, a chocolate milkshake, French fries (which I loved dipping into the milkshake) and two hamburgers - the hamburgers had to be made specially to order so that they were just the burger and the bun. No sauces and even the one possible bit of goodness in the burger - the gherkin - I removed!

As I grew older, attended university and then started work, I continued to be presented with all the usual temptations that surround many of us: socialising, working long hours, commuting, finding time to see friends and family. Who has time to focus on eating well or exercising? Well – no-one. Not unless a change in thinking happens. I realised that there is no point in paying for a gym membership or going on another diet unless the thing that drives all our behaviour - our thoughts - are first evaluated.

And that's what this book is all about. It's about training the mind, so that the body will follow. This book will help you do just that. Consider it a gym of a different sort - *The Thought Gym* – a workout for the mind, with results in the body.

Alarmingly, data (collected in 2008) from the World Health Organisation (WHO) shows that obesity levels have doubled since 1980. Furthermore, 35% of adults are overweight and 11% are obese. These figures are even higher in many Western cultures with percentages in the WHO European Regions indicating that 50% of people are overweight and over 20% are obese. These numbers are expected to rise dramatically in the immediate future. There has been a lot of focus on weight issues and obesity in the media in the last few years and in my opinion, this trend of increasing numbers of people becoming overweight and also obese is the single most important health issue that we will have to face in the coming years. Unhealthy living, consisting of diets high in saturated fats and processed foods, combined with the lack of fresh foods which are high in fibre and nutrients, coupled with not exercising enough, has made being overweight a problem of epidemic proportions. Quite simply put:

> **Unhealthy Living = [Diet High in Saturated Fat] + [Processed Food] – [Fresh food + Exercise]**

The unfortunate reality is that we are sadly lacking the right information on how to live healthy and vibrant lives. Or worse still, we just can't put into practice what we know we *should* be doing. We are bombarded with advertising messages selling us quick-fix foods, quick-fix exercise machines, quick-fix youth and beauty products. We've become a society addicted to quick-fix solutions and dependant on others to solve our problems.

I'm going to let you into a secret now. The fact is... there are no shortcuts in life. In my experience, you always have to pay your dues. Forget the hype about miracle diets or the latest exercise fad in the gym. The simple truth is that in order to achieve and maintain optimum health and fitness, you are going to have to work at it. And keep working at it.

Ok, so that's the bad news. The good news is this. The information in this book will help guide you into making it all seem a lot less like 'work', more like a 'habit' and just part of life. In fact, by the end of it, if you put all of my suggestions into practice, then you won't even realise that you're doing anything special. It will be as natural to you as riding a bike or tying your shoe laces.

I don't believe in diets and I don't believe in rapid weight loss for long term health and happiness. I do appreciate that on the face of it, some of these diets do get results, but ask yourself - *do they really work*? I mean, what's the point of a diet? Is it to lose weight, or to lose weight and keep it off? Have you ever been on a diet? Perhaps it worked at first and then after a few weeks or months you put the weight back on... and then some. If so, you are with the 90% of people that follow diets. They work in the long term less than *10%* of the time. What kind of success rate is that? Would you allow a surgeon to perform an operation on you that only had a 10% success rate? Or get on a plane with a 10% chance of reaching your destination safely? The success rate of diets is appalling and if you continue to jump on the latest diet craze you'll find yourself in a never ending loop. I'll spend time later in the book explaining this, but what you might already recognise is that you are already in (or on the cusp of being in) a perpetual cycle of dieting, weight gain, dieting, and weight gain.

The fact that you have picked up this book is a step in the right direction. It tells me that you're committed to breaking this negative cycle. This book is for you whether you're overweight or just seeking improvements in your weight, physique or health. It's the culmination of my experiences and education over the last 25 years. Many of the techniques in this book come from Neuro-Linguistic Programming (NLP) – a field of human understanding originally created by Dr Richard Bandler and Dr John Grinder in the 1970's, and a brilliant tool for understanding and altering behaviours. I've also drawn inspiration and learnt from other leaders in the fields of human development, health and fitness. There's a section at the end giving you further detail if you want to find out more after finishing this book. Ultimately though, this book is based on my thoughts and experiences around the areas of health and fitness, detailing what I have done to get to where I am today; which is a happy place, where I am in the shape I want to be and feel full of energy. As the chapters unfold, I'll share some of my stories with you so that you come away from reading this book with valuable insights and tools to help you achieve your goals.

Warning!

Only continue reading if:

> ➤ You are committed to making a positive change in your life.
> ➤ You are open minded and willing to take on *and test* new information.
> ➤ You feel that you can be more than you currently are.
> ➤ You're prepared to invest a bit of time and effort into your health and you're not looking for someone to provide you with a quick-fix.

Some of the information in this book you might have seen or heard elsewhere, some of it will be new to you and some of it you might already be doing. And if you're already doing something I describe, then that's great news. It means that we're already on the same page and share similar beliefs, so chances are that you'll like the new stuff too. I just ask that whichever it is, you help yourself and stay committed by keeping an open mind. You don't have to blindly believe everything I present in here. Just take it on board, test it and judge the results for yourself. This book holds valuable concepts that may be the 'difference that makes the difference' for you.

This book has been written in a way that requires interaction – complete interaction between you and me. In other words - you have to *participate*. This is a book to be read actively and then take action. Consider it your journal and confidant. I will be proposing ideas in this book and giving you exercises to complete that will help you on your way. I encourage you to complete them – either in this book (I have left space for your answers) or perhaps in a notebook. The more active you are in the process the greater impact it will have on you and the longer lasting the changes will be.

So, let's take action!

2 –Why?

"He who has a why to live, can bear almost any how." - Friedrich Nietzsche

"Honesty is the first chapter in the book of wisdom" Thomas Jefferson

In order for any of us to do something and to really succeed at it, there has to be a big enough reason *why*. There needs to be a compelling reason as to why *you* are now taking a particular course of action and be honest with yourself about it. Especially if it is going to require a significant portion of your time and energy in order to accomplish it. Even reading this book, I appreciate, is using that most precious of your resources – time. And I thank you for that.

And now it's time to get clear on what your motivations are for embarking on this journey in the first place. Are you unfit and just want to be able to feel energetic each time you play with your kids? Have you decided that it's time to lose that baby weight or want to slim down for your wedding day? We all have our own reasons for losing weight or getting fit. It's time to find out yours and I'm going to help you do this so that you can achieve your goals.

In a moment I will ask you some questions about your motivation and it will be time for you to do as you promised yourself by continuing to read on and participate fully.

To help you along - just in case you need to find some motivation - just think about what being obese, overweight or unhealthy can mean. If you are obese, overweight or otherwise unhealthy then you run a greater risk of:

> Early death   > Cancer
> High blood pressure   > Arthritis
> Diabetes   > Stroke
> Gallbladder disease   > Liver disease
> Kidney disease   > Asthma
> Heart disease   > Back pain

I hope that I've scared you a little and I make no apology for that! I want to stress the importance of being healthy. And in order to do that, you have *got* to remind yourself of what it means to be unhealthy. You will have your own reasons for picking up this book and finally saying "enough is enough!" Let's find out those reasons together.

'MUST' Process

Five reasons why I <u>MUST</u> make _____ happen.

Insert a phrase appropriate for you. For example being fit/being healthier/being 'xx' kilograms. These reasons need to be about something you <u>want</u> rather than something you <u>don't want</u>. So, instead of writing I don't want to huff and puff when I play with my kids; say something like I want to feel vibrant and healthy when I'm playing with my kids. Have a go now.

1) _____

_____

_____

_____

_____

2) _____

_____

_____

_____

_____

3) _____

_____

_____

_____

_____

4) _____

_____

_____

_____

_____

5) _____

_____

_____

_____

_____

Now it's time to up the ante a little. Answer the four questions below. I've given you some examples at the end to help you understand what I mean. There is space for five responses, but feel free to write as much as you can. The more the better, as this process is all about getting you to really be clear on your reasons why you <u>MUST</u> make this change.

1. What <u>will</u> happen if I <u>don't</u> _____?
2. What <u>will</u> happen if I <u>do</u> _____?
3. What <u>won't</u> happen if I <u>do</u> _____?
4. What <u>won't</u> happen if I <u>don't</u> _____?

To assist you with answering the questions above and to get you thinking before you start this exercise here are some examples that people I've helped sometimes give.

Example Answers

Question 1: What <u>will</u> happen if I <u>don't</u> become a healthy weight?

> ➤ I will continue to get fatter and fatter
> ➤ I will need to buy larger clothes
> ➤ I will run a greater risk of developing diabetes
> ➤ I will continue to feel tired and sluggish
> ➤ I will be afraid to go on a beach holiday
> ➤ I will be more susceptible to heart disease

Question 2: What <u>will</u> happen if I <u>do</u> become a healthy weight?

> ➤ I will feel more confident
> ➤ I will be able to enjoy beach holidays again
> ➤ My illnesses will go away
> ➤ My immune system will improve
> ➤ My sex life will improve
> ➤ I will be able to play with the kids more often

Question 3: What <u>won't</u> happen if I <u>do</u> become a healthy weight?

> ➢ I won't be forced to wear baggy clothes any more
> ➢ I won't feel like I'm the worst player on the pitch
> ➢ I won't have to think about whether I can do something or not because of my weight
> ➢ I won't be as likely to develop diseases and illnesses related to my weight
> ➢ I won't be given higher premiums from insurance companies because of my health
> ➢ I won't feel like I need to buy an outfit I don't like as much just because it fits better

Question 4: What <u>won't</u> happen if I <u>don't</u> become a healthy weight?

> ➢ I won't find a partner
> ➢ I won't be able to participate in that charity hike at work
> ➢ I won't be able to play with my grandkids as much
> ➢ I won't have energy to work a full day and then pursue my passion in the evening
> ➢ I won't be able to go on that adventure holiday my partner wants to
> ➢ I won't look as good in my wedding photos

These are just examples to get you thinking and I'm not claiming they will be true for you – they are just listed to get your brain thinking along the right track. The important thing is not whether or not they are true for the masses but that *you* believe them to be true. You need to get leverage on yourself in order to make this (or any) change. And by leverage I mean that taking this action becomes a <u>MUST</u>.

Many people I meet say things like "I should lose weight" or "I ought to exercise more" and "I would like to be healthier" and "I need to eat less". All of those phrases are pointless. Until you are able to change all your *'shoulds', 'ought to's', 'like to's', 'need to's'* and any other phrases like that into a <u>MUST</u>, then the chances are that you won't change.

This is why this step is so important. In order for you to change, you <u>MUST</u> have that compelling reason (or reasons). It must become an absolute <u>MUST</u> for you and I suggest that you stop reading any further until you complete this exercise.

Question 1: What <u>will</u> happen if I <u>don't</u> _____?

1) _____

_____

_____

_____

_____

2) _____

_____

_____

_____

_____

3) _____

_____

_____
_____
_____

4) _____
_____
_____
_____
_____

5) _____
_____
_____
_____
_____

Question 2: What <u>will</u> happen if I <u>do</u> _____?

1) _____
_____
_____
_____
_____

2) _____
_____
_____

_____

_____

3) _____

_____

_____

_____

_____

4) _____

_____

_____

_____

_____

5) _____

_____

_____

_____

_____

Question 3: What <u>won't</u> happen if I <u>do</u> _____?

1) _____

_____

_____

_____

_____

2) _____
_____
_____
_____
_____

3) _____
_____
_____
_____
_____

4) _____
_____
_____
_____
_____

5) _____
_____
_____
_____
_____

Question 4: What <u>won't</u> happen if I <u>don't</u> _____?

1) _____
_____
_____
_____
_____

2) _____
_____
_____
_____
_____

3) _____
_____
_____
_____
_____

4) _____
_____
_____
_____
_____

5) _____
_____

_____

_____

_____

Phew!

Now that the hard part is over, let's be optimistic and write down answers to the following question. Again I've given an example at the beginning of the process to guide you on your way.

Question: Why I know that I <u>CAN</u> change/do this and succeed?

Example responses:

> ➤ I have succeeded in many other areas of my life
> ➤ I love challenges
> ➤ I have this book! ☺
> ➤ I have the support of my family and friends
> ➤ I have a compelling reason why I MUST change
> ➤ I know more now than I did last year

Again, these are just examples. Have fun with it. Remember your past successes – this is not the time to be bashful, so let your ego run wild.

'Why I Can' Process

Question: Why I <u>CAN</u> change/do this and succeed?

1) _____

_____

_____

_____

_____

2) _____

_____

_____

_____

_____

3) _____

_____

_____

_____

_____

4) _____

_____

_____

_____

_____

5) _____

_____

_____

_____

_____

OK, so in this chapter you've now found your 'why', listed all the things that will/won't happen if you do/don't change, and listed why you will succeed. That gives us a good foundation to continue with the rest of the book and the concepts introduced in it. By now, because of the compelling reasons that you've listed, your mind (like this book) should be nicely laid open and ready to receive - if not yet accept - what I'm about to share with you.

Chapter Summary

✓ The most important thing to consider when setting a goal is to discover a big enough 'why' for *why* you are doing it in the first place. Then the 'how' will come.

✓ You wrote down five reasons why you MUST change.

✓ You asked yourself a series of questions to get that reason to be compelling enough.

➢ What will happen if I don't _____?

➢ What will happen if I do _____?

➢ What won't happen if I do _____?

➢ What won't happen if I don't _____?

✓ You also wrote down all the evidence for why you know that you CAN change, by looking at other areas of your life where you have made changes and succeeded.

3 – The Diet Delusion

"The definition of insanity is doing the same thing over and over and over and over again, but expecting a different result." – Albert Einstein

"The rest of the world lives to eat, while I eat to live." - Socrates

Let's get into the substance of this book with something that the 'diet industry' doesn't want you to know, but that you already *do* know. And that is – that, *diets don't work.* And to be clear, when I write the word diet here, I mean any temporary food consumption process which you undertake for rapid and speedy weight loss.

The government recommends a daily calorific intake of 2000 calories for women and 2500 calories for men. Obviously this doesn't take into account size, age, how active you are and several other factors, but for my purposes and the purposes of our goals, this general guideline will do.

Diet books (and this isn't one of them), slimming shakes, weight-loss clubs, weight-loss bars and all the other paraphernalia to do with the weight-loss industry is a multi-billion pound market. From your high protein and low carb diets to your low fat, no fat or no carb diets, it seems as though there are as many different diets out there as ideas for fancy new names. I'll admit that in the short term, some of these diets do help you to lose weight. But, by and large the vast majority of people who complete these diets put the weight straight back on again once the diet is over....and then some more on top too. Moreover, a vast amount of money has been made from the array of diet programs out there – and even if what they claim does work, if your mind isn't right then the program won't work for you anyway. Remember, if you *'train the mind...the body will follow*™'.

So why does dieting often lead to a rebound gain in weight after a short term weight loss? Well, when you undertake a calorie restricted diet, your body doesn't get the number of calories that it might be used to and so while in the short term, it might help with weight loss, when you start eating again (a sensible amount of calories) the body will start to hoard them. This is because in a calorie deprived mode, the body triggers what is known as the 'starvation response' and starts to retain food rather than burn it for fuel. This is because the body is smart - having evolved over thousands of years - and as it doesn't know where the next meal is coming from, it decides to protect itself by keeping hold of the food. In addition, rapid weight loss is often the result of a loss of water from the body and not the quantity of fat you have.

Think about the 'starvation response' for a minute. You (or rather human beings in general - perhaps not you or I) can go months without food. The reason for this is that as food becomes more and more scarce to us, the body with all its remarkable abilities starts to slow down the rate at which it burns calories. You see, many years ago, our ancestors had to cope with droughts, floods, not finding food day to day or hour to hour (unlike us today) and so the body had to survive and the starvation response was the solution. Unfortunately for us, the body can't tell the difference between dieting and starvation and so it unleashes its defence mechanisms.

A calorie is the energy that's needed to raise the temperature of one gram of water by one degree Celsius.

A kilo calorie (kcal or C) is 1000 calories and is what is used on food packaging to denote the amount of energy provided. So, when I say that the average man needs about 2500 calories, it really means 2500 kcal (or 2500 x 1000 calories).

Here are some reasons to stay away from low calorie diets:

1) Low calorie diets will reduce your metabolic rate. Your metabolic rate is the rate at which you can burn off fuel. In essence, the less you eat, the less you burn, the more you eat, the more you burn. It's like when you adjust your spending to suit your budget. When I finished university, I went off travelling. While travelling, I lived on just over £100 a week and I was able to get by quite happily with that. When I returned home and started working, I was earning £400 a week and my lifestyle changed in accordance with that, as I started to spend according to my means. When I lost that job through redundancy, I was suddenly on an allowance from the government and had to live on £60 a week. Do you think that my lifestyle changed a bit? Was I able to go out and live as I had or did my rate of living have to slow down? You bet it did. And it's the same with your metabolism. The less food in, the slower your metabolism is in order to adjust. Your metabolism is not fixed and changes with aging and what you do and what you eat. Things like exercising boosts your metabolism, as does adding chilli to your meal, as does drinking water and eating little and often. The excuse of 'having a slow metabolism' won't work with me – sorry!

In fact, when calories are restricted you can slow your metabolism by 20-30% and even more in extreme cases. This is all well documented in other books and so I'm not going to dwell on it, but it's hopefully got you realising that calorie restricted diets aren't the answer.

2) In addition, low calorie diets also cause a lot of the weight loss to come from muscle and not fat, and with others it is water weight that you are losing. They also increase the activity of the enzymes responsible for storing fat but reduce those responsible for burning fat. Furthermore, low calorie diets decrease the output from your thyroid hormone which is responsible for regulation of your basal metabolic rate - the rate at which you burn fat for fuel.

Have you ever been on a diet only to find out that when you came off it, you put all of the weight back on and then more too? Initially, when you're on the diet, things look like they're going well. The diet is working and you're losing weight and then you hit a plateau (largely as your body adapts to the reduction in calories as described above). You then start to get a little despondent about not getting the results you were getting and then you start to eat something that you shouldn't and then before you know it, you're eating what you were before but only this time, because your body has been in starvation mode, it continues to hoard the food. Your metabolism has already reduced, so although you're eating the same as what you did before, you actually find that you put on more weight.

So then what do you do? You try another diet, and so the cycle starts again, and again, and again. Before you know it, you're in this endless loop of diet after diet. That's no way to live, in my opinion. Better to stick to eating a food regime that is sensible, sustainable and one that you enjoy.

And even if you're not on a calorie restricted diet, but one a bit like the Atkins diet which restricts food types, then that's just as bad, if not even worse. High fat diets and low fat diets alike are not the answer. Sensible sizes, around 20% of your dietary intake should be from fats – and the good type, like the polyunsaturated fats found in fish, nuts, seeds and leafy greens. Stay away from as many saturated fats as possible found in food like meat, butter, cream, cheese, eggs and full fat yogurt. The only way for you to really stay healthy is if you adopt a habit of sensible healthy eating which you can maintain for a lifetime. Forget the never ending cycle of quick-fix dieting which is unsustainable in the long term.

OK, so what are the other reasons why diets don't work? I mentioned the word 'temporary' and the majority of these diets provide exactly that – a temporary fix. The goal of most diets, especially those with unrealistic expectations about which foods you can and can't eat is this; it's to get you to your target weight but they don't think beyond that. The goal for many of these diet books is for you to attain but not *maintain* your target weight.

This is a good point to introduce you to the concept of the unconscious mind (or sub-conscious mind, as it's sometimes referred to). Most of us are familiar with the concept of having a conscious mind – the part of the mind which makes all the conscious decisions – like "what should I wear today?" or "what shall I cook?" The unconscious mind is responsible for a whole host of other things like regulating your body temperature, making sure you breathe, organising your memories and making mental associations. Your unconscious mind is actually massively more powerful and active to your well-being than you probably realise. Think of your whole mind (conscious and unconscious) as being like an iceberg. You could consider that the tip of the iceberg; the thing we actually notice, is the conscious mind, but what supports that, below the surface and many times larger, is the massive remainder of the iceberg – the unconscious mind.

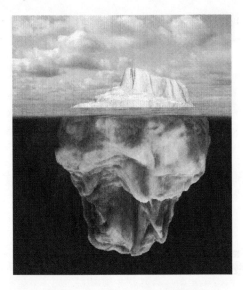

When you consider just how large and prominent the unconscious mind is, you begin to appreciate that perhaps what goes into that unconscious mind is very important. Studies into the power of the unconscious mind are really only in their infancy and it's quite exciting where this field of research is going to lead. But getting back to the task in hand; when you consciously set a diet as a goal, it becomes set in the unconscious mind too. It understands it's on a 6-week diet (or whatever the length of time happens to be), but it also understands that it's just *temporary*.

I consider diets to be a lot like projects. By that I mean that a project is something with a goal, a timeline for achieving it and a method (or strategy) for getting there. Imagine this scenario for a moment. It's two months until barbeque season and you want your garden to look great for a party. You get a plan together including: deciding what needs to happen and when, hiring a gardener and then overseeing the project. Two months pass and you have a fabulous garden - ready to entertain all your friends. What happens though once the party is over, now that the goal has been achieved? If you want the garden to remain looking nice, you're going to have to make sure that you have all the right tools and strategies in place to maintain it. Otherwise without the right tools and appropriate effort, the lawn will overgrow, the weeds will take over and your path will get covered in moss. And diets are similar, in that they have a goal, timeline and strategy for getting there. The trouble is that their goal is usually just to get you to the size/weight/physique you want and not provide you with the skills, tools and mindset that you need to maintain what you've achieved. And when you've achieved your goal, your unconscious mind realises this also and says: "So – now what?" and it moves its focus from the target to shift its attention elsewhere. If there are no plans in place with how to continue along the healthy route then all your effort is wasted. The start of any goal should really be to hit your target weight, get into that outfit or be that perfect shape. Then the *real* goal (and it's an ongoing one) is to maintain and improve upon it. It's really important to be thinking in those terms and not just looking 2, 4, 6 weeks into the future - only seeing yourself at a particular party or on a particular beach and not seeing yourself beyond that point in time. Your unconscious mind needs the message from you that this is the way it is from now on - not just that this is how it is for the short term only. After all, there are going to be many more barbeques and it's better to maintain that garden consistently instead of having to start from scratch each and every time.

So start right now to get into the mindset of a lifestyle diet, one with healthy unprocessed foods and remove from your consciousness the idea of following the next new fangled diet that some celebrity is endorsing. Trust me, in the long term it's better to take small steps to get there and *stay* there, rather than just following a diet plan which offers quick large gains. It's not healthy to have your body change that dramatically and quickly anyway and it won't work in the long run.

Chapter Summary

- ✓ Diets don't work. And you know this because you've *tried* many in the past and none have lasted.
- ✓ When you limit your food, your body adapts to trigger its starvation response leading it to retain whatever food it gets and not burn it off.
- ✓ Lowering your calorific intake reduces your metabolic rate.
- ✓ Your unconscious (or subconscious) mind plays an important role in all that you do.
- ✓ Diets are short term and don't cater for the long term approach to health and well-being.

4 – Beliefs

"Whatever the mind of man can conceive and believe, he can achieve." – Napoleon Hill

"The only way of finding the limits of the possible is by going beyond them into the impossible." – Arthur C. Clarke

What are beliefs? I'm not speaking about religious beliefs here. Beliefs are the rules of our lives; emotionally held opinions which are treated by us as fact. They can be empowering such as "I am a great presenter" or limiting like "I'll never be good at cooking". These beliefs - the rules to our lives, have the power to transform us for better or for worse.

We form our beliefs in three ways. As the result of our own direct experience, the experience of others relayed to us and experiences we observe. For example, I could touch a hot stove and know not to do it in the future, or someone else could have done it in the past and tell me not to touch it, or I could witness someone else do it and realise not to do it. These experiences are then interpreted by us and ultimately shape our beliefs around things. Often we might generalise an experience and apply it to all situations – a 'global' belief. For example, you might have had a nasty experience with a door-to-door salesperson and generalise that all salespeople are like that. Will that affect how you answer the door to the next door-to-door salesperson? My assumption is that it will. As Shakespeare wrote – "nothing is good or bad, but thinking makes it so."

So, what about beliefs about yourself? If you believe that you won't succeed at turning your health, energy or weight issues around, do you think you'll succeed? Of course not! You see, our minds don't like to be proved wrong and we will do whatever we can to confirm an expectation or belief that we have. The mind will look for ways to substantiate your point – it's not a case of we believe what we see, more that *we see what we believe*. As Henry Ford is quoted as saying, "If you think you can, or you think you can't, either way you're right". There's a story about when Henry Ford once asked his engineers to build a V8 engine. Now I'm pretty useless when it comes to cars, so I couldn't even tell you what a V8 is! Suffice it to say, it might be commonplace now, but back then it was unheard of to put this amount of power into one car. His engineers said it couldn't be done, and sure enough, six months later, they came back and proved it couldn't. Undeterred, Ford insisted that they build this thing and another six months went by with nothing. Henry Ford told his engineers that no matter what it takes, they were to figure out a way to build one as he believed it could be done, even if they didn't and sure enough, they eventually did. Now do you think that had Ford been swayed by the beliefs of his engineers that this would ever have been achieved? I bet not.

What about Roger Bannister? Previous to him, no one in history had succeeded in running a mile in under four minutes. Then in 1954 Roger Bannister succeeded where all others before him had failed. How did he do this? Well aside from undertaking a lot of physical and mental rehearsal, he held a belief; a strong unshakeable belief that it could be done. And he was right. He ran it in 3 minutes 59 seconds. What is even more remarkable is that the same year, more athletes then broke the 4 minute barrier and the following year there were dozens more that did. Was it a change in their fitness, training, diet or technology in that short period of time that made this possible? No. The only thing that changed for them was the belief that it could be done. History is rich with examples of people achieving the seemingly impossible and it's all down to what they *believed* was possible for them.

We don't all want to build high performance vehicles or run four minute miles, but we might want to look at some of the beliefs that we currently hold and whether or not they are serving us. We have a personal investment in our beliefs. When the world validates our beliefs, things make sense to us; we feel secure and understand what's going on. As soon as something comes along to challenge our beliefs we become unsure and doubtful. If that old belief of ours gets replaced with a new belief, it usually changes our whole outlook. And if you don't believe me, just think back to when you were a child and believed in Father Christmas or the Tooth Fairy. Or perhaps more recently in getting a job or promotion you once didn't believe you could get. Perhaps it was something else for you? All of us have had times in our lives when a belief we had in something was altered by something that happened. What happened to your view of the world when those beliefs were changed? Changing our beliefs can be one of the most powerful ways to change how we live in the world.

Let's do a couple of processes now. They're going to require you to form some pictures in your mind, so before we get into the processes properly, let's just warm up first. Some people I work with say that they have difficulty in visualising or forming pictures in their minds. The truth is that we can all do it. Just think for a second. What does your front door look like? Does it open to the left or the right? What posters did you have on your wall at home when you were a teenager? In order for you to answer these questions – even if it was with an "I don't know", required that you had some pictorial representation of it in your mind – an image. Even looking in the mirror requires that you have an image in your head about what you look like – otherwise it would be as if you were an amnesia sufferer every time you looked in the mirror! If you've seen the movie *'Momento'*, you know what I mean.

Let's get back to the main process now. Read through the entire process first before doing it so that you understand what you have to do. Read until the part which says: **'now go back to the beginning of this process and have a go yourself'.**

Belief Identification Process

Write down a belief that you feel is limiting you. For example

> ➢ "No pain, no gain"
> ➢ "I can't get what I want"
> ➢ "I can't work a computer"

In your case perhaps something to do with the reason for picking up this book, like

> ➢ "I never stick to working out"
> ➢ "I always quit when the going gets tough"

Fill in your answers below

a) Limiting belief:

_____

_____

_____

_____

Now write down a belief that you used to believe but now don't. Perhaps it is something about Father

Christmas, or the Tooth Fairy, perhaps you once believed you could never run a marathon but did it, or go travelling by yourself but then went exploring on your own.

b) Old belief:

_____

_____

_____

_____

Now write down a positive belief that you want to have instead of the limiting one in step (a). Maybe it's something along the lines of "I am able to make healthy food choices".

c) Positive belief:

_____

_____

_____

_____

Now write down a belief that you are absolutely certain about; like the sun will rise tomorrow, the seasons change, the sun rises in the east and sets in the west.

d) Belief you are certain about:

_____

_____

_____

_____

Belief Change Process

Read this entire process first to get a feel for it before attempting it. For guided support please go to: http://thethoughtgym.com/book

For this process, it's important not to over think the process but allow the answers to come almost without thinking. The key to this process is speed and you must answer the questions quickly. I recommend asking a friend to do this with you or using the guided materials.

1. Okay, for whatever you answered for belief in (a) above, I want you to bring an image of it to your mind as you think about this belief. Something will appear; something that represents that belief for you.

2. Use the table provided on the following page to answer questions about the image. As you think about the image, in a moment, you will need to note down the responses that result after being asked the question in step 3. Note the answer under the correct column (in this case for belief (a)). Use just a letter to abbreviate the answer as the questions must be asked quickly (e.g. 'B' for black & white, 'N' for near etc). If you are working with a friend, ask them to ask the questions and make a note of your responses.

3. So, getting back to the image. Allow that image to come to your mind and answer the following questions about it.

Is the image........?

	Belief (a)	Belief (b)	Belief (c)	Belief (d)
B & W or Colour				
Near or Far				
Bright or Dim				
Location (is it in front, to the side)				
Size (big, small, huge etc)				
Associated (own eyes) **or Disassociated** (see yourself in picture)				
Framed or Panoramic				
Movie or Still				
Many images or just one				
[Movie] Fast/Normal/Slow				
3D or Flat				
Viewing angle (above, side, below...)				

4. Now think of something completely different – think about where you last went on holiday, or who is number one in the charts right now. (I'll refer to this as 'breaking state' later on – i.e. When I ask you to think of something completely different.)

5. Now do step 1 - 3 again but with the old belief you used to hold, belief (b). Notice everything about that image as you did before. Colour, size, location, movie/still, contrasts etc and put these in the column under (b).

6. Break your state again – think about something completely different. What was the last book you read? Who's your favourite actor?

7. Notice the big differences between the two images. Was one black and white, while the other colour? In one of the pictures were you looking through your own eyes but in the other you could see yourself in it? Was one up close to you but the other far away? One a movie but the other a still image? Notice the biggest differences that you had. Perhaps circle them.

8. Now here's the fun part. Bring the image from belief (a) to your attention and start to play with the qualities of that image. Make the image take on qualities from the second image; your belief (b). For example, if the image you had for belief (a) was colour but the image you had for belief (b) was black and white, I want you to make the image for belief (a) black and white as well. The same with the location. Move belief (a) to where belief (b) was

positioned and make it a similar size. Anything that was distinctly different between the two images I want you to transfer the quality from the limiting belief image in (a) to make it like the belief in (b).

9. Break your state. What does your front door look like? Does it open to the right, or to the left?

10. Now, similarly, with the new positive belief that you wrote down for belief (c) – bring all the qualities of the image to life as you did before (steps 1 – 3). Notice the image you have - its size, location, colour, contrast, whether it's a movie or still image, how many pictures. Go down the table and notice the qualities. If you're doing this with a friend, ask them to read out the different qualities quickly, almost allowing you no time to think. Call out the answers and get them to note them down under column (c).

11. Break your state and think of something else. What's your favourite book? Which book did you read most recently?

12. Now bring to your mind an image that represents belief (d) and take note of all the qualities of that image. Size, colour, location etc as listed in the table above. Again, do this quickly and make a note under column (d).

13. Break your state and think of something else. What was the last mode of transport you took?

14. Notice all the major differences between the results under columns (c) and (d). Perhaps circle them. For example, one might have been in 3D but the other 2D. One colour, the other black and white.

15. Now bring back to your mind the image you had for belief (c) and start to change the qualities of that image to become like those in belief (d). For example, if the image of your desired positive belief from belief (c) was in the bottom right of your field of view and in black and white and small, but the image you held for belief (d) was full colour and in front of you on a gigantic screen, then move the image from belief (c) to look like that.

This may take a bit of getting used to and I advise you to perform it in pairs of beliefs. I.e. first do beliefs (a) & (b) – steps 1- 9, and then move on to beliefs (c) & (d), steps 10 - 15.

If you're working on your own, make sure that you understand and have remembered the process so you don't have to break your concentration to focus on what is needed next.

If you have a partner with you then they can assist by asking you the questions of what the image looks like.

Again, if you need help with this process and don't have a partner to help you, then please go to http://thethoughtgym.com/book for a guided walk-through of this process. OK, if you're ready, now go **back to the beginning of this process and have a go for yourself**.

How did you get on? How does the belief seem different to you right now? Does the limiting belief seem less real now? Does the positive belief you want see like it's a bit clearer now, or more certain? If you need to go back and practise some more, then go right ahead.

The reason that beliefs are so important in your quest for a better you is that they really do shape your reality. If you truly believe that you'll never be thin, then, guess what? That's exactly what your reality will end up being for you. Like I said before, but I'll repeat it again here for emphasis. Our mind will do what it can to prove ourselves right. If we say we can or we can't do something then both our conscious and our unconscious mind will work to validate that statement.

The way your unconscious mind works is a bit like a computer. You ask it a question and it will go off behind the scenes to find the answer for you – even working on it when you are doing something else – it's the original multi-tasker!

To illustrate - imagine you come up against a particular challenge at work or home. Let's say that you want to go on an adventure holiday for three weeks and so need that time off work. Scenario A has you believing that it will never happen and inside (even though you may not even be conscious of it) you believe that it won't be OK with your boss so you say to yourself:

> ➤ *"I don't think my boss is going to allow me to take that much time off"*

Your little computer program will go off searching for all the reasons why that statement is right. He rejected someone else's leave, it's near the financial year-end or you have a huge workload on.

Whereas, let's present another scenario B where you believe that you will be able to go and so you ask yourself:

> ➢ *"How do I need to approach this so that I get to go?"*

You are more likely to come up with better answers such as - I can organise my workload or clients before or after the trip, I can catch him on a good day and highlight the fact I've never taken this type of leave, although it is near the financial year-end, my team has been well trained to handle it in my absence.

I hope you get the idea with that one. The beliefs that you hold about yourself, your environment or the people you meet will shape how you think and behave. What the process described above can do - and it's something I didn't know until a few years ago - is that you don't have to wait for something to change a belief for you; you can influence it and indeed initiate a change of belief by yourself. Sounds simple? Well, it is!

The power of being able to change your beliefs will literally change how you interact with the world around you and as a direct consequence it will change what you are capable of doing. In order for the world around you to change, first YOU must change.

Chapter Summary

- ✓ Beliefs are rules that govern how we run our lives.
- ✓ Beliefs can be empowering or limiting.
- ✓ You wrote down a limiting belief that you held about exercise or health.
- ✓ You worked through a process to change that limiting belief into something more positive.

5 - Values

"We do not act rightly because we have virtue or excellence, but we rather have those because we have acted rightly." – Aristotle

"It's not hard to make decisions when you know what your values are." - Roy Disney

What are your values? Let's start by asking – *what is a value?* A value is really a determining factor or standard that you use to make your choices in life and once you understand what they are, you can influence and change your choices. They can act as filters on our world so that we only pay attention to the things we value. They can act as decision makers and influence how we will behave and act in certain situations.

There is a straightforward process that you can use to determine what your values are in any situation. And it's really the answer to the following question.

What's important to me in 'X'?

Replace 'X' with what you want to find your values in. For example: life, work, family, vacations, education, health and so forth.

For the purposes of our work together and making the assumption that you want to change your physique, weight or some other aspect of your health I will use something related to health as an example.

In fact, in order to really get stuck into this process, we really need to ask ourselves two very similar questions.

    A.   *What's important to me in 'life'?*

    B.   *What's important to me in 'exercise'* (or health, fitness, physique etc)?

Question (A) I recommend answering as it is written, but for question (B) change the word 'exercise' for something else appropriate to your goal like 'my weight', 'my physique', 'my health'.

Don't answer just yet, as there's a process for this. You will answer the questions listing what those mean to you. Also, let me just point out that the values need to be 'ends' values and not 'means' values. An example of a 'means' value would be money, or family or relationship – but what do those things give you in the 'end'? Is it security, love, connection?

Values Identification Process

So the process will be like this:

1) Take a sheet of A4 paper and write down the question at the top of the paper (this will help you keep focused).

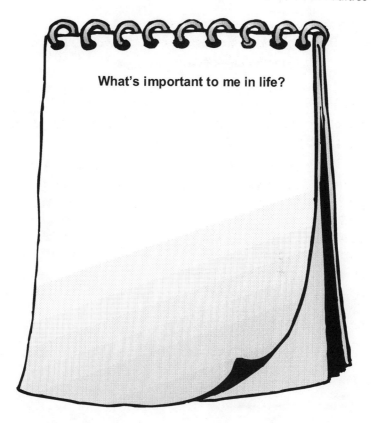

What's important to me in life?

2) Then list all the values that you hold for that question along the left hand side with space left next to the value to write what belief you hold about that value.

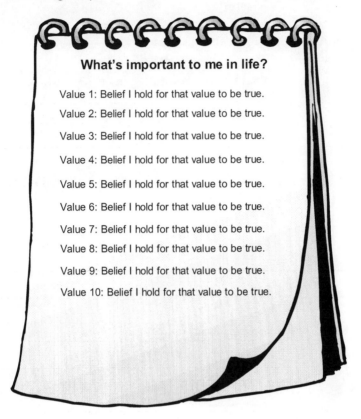

What's important to me in life?

Value 1: Belief I hold for that value to be true.

Value 2: Belief I hold for that value to be true.

Value 3: Belief I hold for that value to be true.

Value 4: Belief I hold for that value to be true.

Value 5: Belief I hold for that value to be true.

Value 6: Belief I hold for that value to be true.

Value 7: Belief I hold for that value to be true.

Value 8: Belief I hold for that value to be true.

Value 9: Belief I hold for that value to be true.

Value 10: Belief I hold for that value to be true.

The reason that you need to write both the value *and* the belief you hold for it is because two people might have the same values - so for example they might both put 'love' as a top value in life, but what they *believe* about love is different. One person might recognise love as when someone does small intimate things for the other, but the other person may believe that love is when they are showered with gifts all the time.

So what you need to do is write your value along the left and then write your belief about that value (i.e.

what you need in order to have that value satisfied), next to it on the right.

The format for writing your values will then look like this:

Value	**Belief** – i.e. what must happen in order for that value be true for you

3) Then, cut the paper into strips so there is one value and belief per strip. E.g.

Value 1	**Belief** – i.e. what must happen in order for that value be true for you

Value 2	**Belief** – i.e. what must happen in order for that value be true for you

Value 3	**Belief** – i.e. what must happen in order for that value be true for you

4) The next task will be to order or prioritise those values. Look at your list of values and choose the one that you could do without – your *least* important one. And place that to one side. So, if you have a list of [10] values – ask yourself which one of them you would lose if you really had to. That then goes to the bottom of the new list. Then, for the [9] remaining values, ask yourself which one of those you would lose if you had to. Place that one above the first one you originally moved to the new list. Continue to do this until you have a prioritized list of [10] values.

For example:

Value 8	**Belief** – i.e. what must happen in order for that value be true for you

Value 4	**Belief** – i.e. what must happen in order for that value be true for you

Value 2	**Belief** – i.e. what must happen in order for that value be true for you

And so on. In the example above, the priority order is this:

Priority	**Value Number** (as written down when first listing them)
1	8
2	4
3	2

Here is an example of some of mine from when I first completed the process.

Question

What's important to me in 'life'?

1) **Health:** 12% body fat, run 10k in under 40 minutes, no aches and pains
2) **Security:** Mortgage free, access to money, high level of healthcare available, having capabilities to control my outcomes

3) **Respect:** Having opinion valued, helping others, being honest

4) **Love:** Do anything for someone, supports me unconditionally, little treats/acts of kindness or caring

And so on. I did this process in 2006 and I had 12 listed in all. Now what was interesting when doing this process again in 2011 was that although the values were largely the same and roughly in the same order, my beliefs about what it took to satisfy those values were different.

My top value for health from 2006 was not realistic in its entirety. I had never managed a 10k run in under 40 minutes and I constantly had a few aches and pains. Now for me to define having health as that meant I was always going to be coming up short. In 2011, I noticed that my definition for health had changed to read:

"I feel healthy when I'm able to do any physical activity I want to and I'm able to do it freely and with ease."

That's a fair bit easier for me to meet and I feel more content because of it. Now, you could argue that that's less to do with health and more to do with fitness, but the point is this. When you come to do this process, understanding how you define your values will determine whether or not you feel you will ever be able to meet them.

Here are some examples of how someone might answer the second question. The second question was:

What's important to me in exercise?

You could have:

1) **Variety**: Doing a number of different disciplines or classes

2) **Company**: Exercising with friends, colleagues or in a class

3) **Recognition**: Getting a medal
4) **Challenge**: Something only few people achieve
5) **Effectiveness**: Will see measurable and big results in less than 4 weeks
6) **Enjoyment**: Makes me laugh, time goes by quickly, feels relaxing
7) **Cost**: Is cheap or free, worth every penny
8) **Equipment**: Lots of equipment needed, or lots of latest gadgets involved
9) **Local**: Can travel within 10 minutes of work/home

Ok, if you think you've got this, put the book down and take as much time as you need to do this exercise now, and then come back to the book. To help you with this, or for more guidance, please go to http://thethoughtgym.com/book for the guided version.

.... Ok, have you done it?

No?

Well, go back and do it!

Right, by now I believe that you've done it. What did you notice about your answers to those two questions? How do your values help or hinder you? Did you have success listed as your top value, or adventure or fun? Where was health on the list? Was it up in the top one or two? Top five? If it was any lower than the top 1 or 2, we need to do something about that. Why? What if you have love (i.e. for your family), or success (work, family, social life) at the top of your list? Would you really be able to fully meet any of those values if health wasn't a priority? Could you look after your family, could you have as much fun or adventure? Could you endure the long hours needed to be successful? Could you contribute as much if you were unwell or limited by your health or fitness?

I suggest to you that if health is not high up on your list, then you won't make it a priority and you're likely to suffer because of it. Perhaps what got you to pick this book up in the first place was that you didn't have health as a high enough priority and you do now? I'm assuming that for the majority, health doesn't appear that high up in the ordered list.

What can we do about this then? Is there a way to move the value at priority 7 on the list above the one at priority 1? Why is it important to know how we organise our values?

Well, the fact that you now have awareness about your values is a *massive* step forward. When I discovered what my values were it made a big difference to my understanding about how I made my decisions. For the most part, my decisions were based on whether my actions would meet the highest values. If they did, I was more likely to carry out the action. I'll give you an example – I like to walk. In fact, I prefer walking around the city rather than getting on public transport. By default it meets my two highest values - I get to exercise (meeting the health one) and I don't spend money unnecessarily (meeting security and financial).

I remember once when I used to work for a corporate company, a colleague and I needed to go from one office to the other for a meeting. It just started to rain and so for my colleague, Richard, his instinctive action was to hail a cab (bear in mind that we're only talking about a 10-15 minute walk and a cab in London would take just as long). I had already taken an umbrella with me and the idea of a cab, or even getting the tube (as others often did) didn't even enter my mind. You see, in that context at least, Richard was more concerned about getting wet and dishevelled than he was about paying £10 for being stuck in traffic in the back of a cab. He placed a higher value on appearance or comfort than I did. I also realised that this was perhaps why I cycled to work each day, and he did not, despite him always saying that he wanted to. He would have to carry his bike up a flight of stairs to his flat (not comfortable), wear a helmet (perceived by him not to look good or fashionable), wear some kind of day-glow outfit (urgh!!) and the rest. Whereas, I figured that cycling was economical, healthy and a more reliable form of transport. In other words cycling met my health value by working out, was cheaper than travelling on public transport (security/money) and I was also guaranteed to know when I would arrive at work each day. In addition, I would not be at the mercy of the notorious London transport system (also meeting my security value – having the capability to affect my outcome).

Here's the interesting thing though.   Once I realised just how I was basing my decisions, I was able to better evaluate whether that was the right approach. To give you an example, I wanted more adventure and risk-taking in my life and wanted to go sky-diving but it cost quite a lot and security (of finances) was a value I prioritized above adventure and risk-taking. However to fulfil my goal of sky-diving I realised that I would have to (at least temporarily) press a 'pause' button on the values above the 'adventure' and 'risk-taking' values. If I always made decisions unconsciously based on how my values were organised, without the awareness of actually how I organised them, I would be restricting my decision-making ability.   This would affect what experiences I would have and ultimately affect the quality of my life. The sheer fact that I now have an *awareness* on how I base my decisions, means that I am now more free to choose and more importantly, able to control my choices rather than letting those choices remain automatic to me. I've used this to great effect in the last few years. One such example was back in 2009 when I decided to go to Everest Base Camp. The trip was, as I discovered, going to be expensive. I could have put that money to use elsewhere, but I also had a passion for adventure, learning and growing – albeit further down on the list than security. As I was aware of this, I was able to suspend that value temporarily (realising it was inhibiting me) and meet my need for adventure, learning and growing.

I touched on this earlier but a second way to deal with the values and make them work for you is to understand what you have to believe in order for that value to be true. Could they be re-defined to make them fit in with your goals? Take one of mine as an example. I already mentioned that one of my values from 2006 was 'security'.

> **Security**: Mortgage free, access to money, high level of healthcare available, having capabilities to control my outcomes

What if your value was the same – security – but the belief about it was different? For example:

> **Security**: Knowing that I have the resourcefulness and capabilities to deal with whatever situation presents itself to me.

How would something like that be different? Would you be open to new opportunities? Take more action?

A third way to work on the list you have (in addition to having an awareness of them and redefining the belief you hold about particular values) is to change the actual order of them. We can do this by changing how your values are represented in your mind. The following process will do just that. Read it all the way through before doing it, so that you know what to do.

Value Switch Process

1. Think of a value which is one that you would like to have higher up on your list. For example, you might have 'health' or 'fitness' at number 8 or 9, but you have success at number 1. We already mentioned you can't really hope to be successful if you can't look after yourself so you might want to place a higher level of importance on health.

2. What image comes to mind when you think of that value? Perhaps working out in the gym, perhaps waiting in the cold in the school playground before gym class, maybe it's eating beans, or maybe it's the image a loved one who is ill? Think about that image?

3. Is it a positive or a negative one?

4. If it's a negative image then first you'll need to switch the image using a technique I describe after this one, so skip ahead until you see "Swish Pattern" technique.

5. If it's already a positive image, then ask the follow questions and make a note of the answers (just like we did in the belief change process earlier) in the table on the following page, under image 1. Again, you might want to enlist the help of a friend or go to http://thethoughtgym.com/book for help.

Is the image......?

	Image 1	Image 2
B & W or Colour		
Near or Far		
Bright or Dim		
Location (is it in front, to the side)		
Size (big, small, huge etc)		
Associated (own eyes) **or Disassociated** (see yourself in picture)		
Framed or Panoramic		
Movie or Still		
Many images or just one		
[Movie] Fast/Normal/Slow		
3D or Flat		
Viewing angle (above, side, below...)		

6. Now, having made a note of all the qualities - clear your mind ('break state'). Think about where you last went on holiday or where you'd like to go next.

7. Next, think about a value that you have high on the list and in the appropriate position that you'd like to move the first (lower down the list) value you elicited.

8. What image comes to mind for that value?

9. Again make a note of qualities and put them in the column for image 2.

10. Now, clear the mind again. Who was your first crush?

11. What were the biggest differences between the two? Was one black and white, while the other colour? Was one large and vibrant while the other small and far away?

12. Make a note of those biggest differences. Usually it's characteristics like colour, size, associated or not, location.

13. Get the image of the lower down value – the one you want to move up your list.

14. Start to change the image to match more of the qualities of the higher up value.

15. Hold that image for a few seconds and really feel and live it.

16. In what way does it feel differently to you now? Has the value moved further up the list? It might not be

where the other one was, but is it moving in the right direction?

This kind of technique takes a bit of getting used to so go easy on yourself and practise it. It might take a while as it's something new. Go to http://thethoughtgym.com/book for the guided support.

Swish Pattern Technique

If you had a negative image when thinking of the value you need to change, for example, you think of exercise and you see yourself in a gym being overweight and you think that everyone around you is judging you (they're not by the way – that's just your own mind reading into the situation) then this technique can be used to change the image.

It's an NLP process called the Swish Pattern (you'll find out why in a sec) but here's what you need to do. First read it all the way through and perhaps it might be helpful to get someone to do this with you. Closing your eyes to do this process often helps, so be sure to know the steps first or go to http://thethoughtgym.com/book for the guided support.

1. Think of the image that comes to your mind when you think of that value. The negative image. We'll call this the *Present State*.

2. Associate into that image – in other words, if you're not already looking through your own eyes, step into the image and notice how you feel.

3. OK, step out and clear the screen. Open your eyes and think of something else. Who's your favourite author?

4. Now create a new image to match that value but one which is more positive in nature. For example, if your image earlier was the gym and not feeling or looking comfortable in there, change the image to one more inspiring for you like running along the beach feeling really happy.

5. Be fully associated into the image – notice the colours, sounds, feelings that you have.

6. Good, now while maintaining that image, step out of it (i.e. become disassociated so you can see yourself in it and you are not looking through your own eyes). We'll call this the *Desired State*.

7. OK, break your state and think of something else. What was the last movie you went to see?

8. Bring back the Present State image (from steps 1 and 2). Now fully associate back into it.

9. Insert a small dark picture of the desired state from step 6 into the lower left corner of the other image.

10. Make sure you can see yourself in that little image.

11. Now for the swish part.

12. While making a swish sound, simultaneously have your Desired State (the one from step 6) become bigger and brighter while at the same time have your Present State image (from step 1 which represents that value) become small and shrink into nothing in the lower left hand corner.

13. Open your eyes and clear your mind. Think of something else. Who do you most admire?

14. Repeat steps 8 to 13 again, this time a little faster.

15. Keep on repeating steps 8-14, getting faster and faster each time. Do this at least 15 times, remembering to break your state after each time and clear your mind.

Once you've done it at least 15 times, now try and think of that old (un-serving) value and see what image comes to mind. Does the old image appear, or is the change so fast that the new desired image appears? If not, go back and repeat the process until you get it. It takes a bit of practice at first because it's something new and different so persevere. As Pablo Picasso once said "I am always doing that which I cannot do, in order that I may learn how to do it."

For around 20% of people, the image starting from the bottom right hand side of the screen might work better, so experiment a little and see what works for you.

Hopefully now you have a positive image associated to that particular value, you can go back and complete the value switch process on it (if it's not already changed its position in your values list through doing this exercise).

There's been a lot of material and exercises covered in this chapter, so you might want to go back and review it and spend a little time on this before moving on. Remember, your path to health and well-being should be seen by you as an ongoing journey, more like a marathon than a sprint, so there's no point rushing through this book just to get to the end.

Chapter Summary

✓ Values determine how you make choices and act as a filter on the world.

✓ You determined what values you hold important in certain areas of your health and well being.

✓ You listed these values and also what about that value makes it true for you.

✓ Using the process where you examined the qualities of the values, you worked to change the order of these values

✓ You were introduced to the Swish Pattern to change some negative values into more positive one.

6 – Language

"In the course of my life, I have often had to eat my words, and I must confess that I have always found it a wholesome diet." - Winston Churchill

"If you talk to a man in a language he understands, that goes to his head. If you talk to him in his language - that goes to his heart." – Nelson Mandela

Perhaps the greatest influence on how we think about ourselves comes from our own language. What we hear others say to us, about us and most importantly how we talk to ourselves. We are constantly talking to ourselves, whether we like to admit it or not. These can be empowering or disempowering depending on what we say. For instance, when you were buying this book, perhaps you were asking yourself *"Is this worth it?"*; *"will it work for me?"* When you wake up in the morning, you might say something like: *"Uh, is it time to wake up already?"*; *"why do I have to go in to work today?"* Whether it's conscious or not, you are talking to yourself *all the time.*

So this chapter is all about language and how a change in the way we describe experiences actually changes how we *feel* about that experience. As Shakespeare told us, via Hamlet: "There is nothing either good or bad, but thinking makes it so."

I'll start with an example. I used to really not like doing the ironing. It was such a chore. I used to say to myself *"Ah, I HAVE to do the ironing this weekend"*. But when I made one simple change, the way I felt about doing the ironing changed. I simply changed the *'have* to', to a *'want* to'. That was it. You see, the ironing is still going to get done but now how I feel about the whole experience is different. Wouldn't you agree that when you say that you *have* to, *need* to, *ought* to, *should* do something, it feels a lot different in your body than saying that you *want to* do it? Try it. Say a few things now and feel the difference.

I started doing it with a lot of other phrases and I started saying things like I *want* to get up at 6am tomorrow and I *want* to go to the gym. I *want* to do the housework, I *want* to vacuum today. It was such a revelation and so simple!

You can even take things a step further and move the 'want' to a 'will' or 'am' phrase. For example the stages might be

> ➢ I need to get up at 6am to go to the gym (has negative feelings associated with it)

To

> ➢ I *want* to get up at 6am to go to the gym (feelings of want lead you to desire something and will produce different feelings inside you)

To

> ➢ I *am/will be* getting up at 6am tomorrow to go to the gym (this is a statement of certainty – once it's made, it becomes a commitment to the unconscious mind and very difficult to break. Your brain doesn't want to be proved wrong remember).

I personally interchange between want to and am/will, depending on whether I want to create a bit of emotional inspiration, so I might usually say, if I'm in the pub with my friends and I'm not drinking (which is often the case) and they encourage me to have a pint or something, then I will usually say that I *want* to get up early the next morning and so can't. If I say to myself I want to go to the gym, I start to get more excited about the whole experience. It's important to have this feeling of desire as it implies that there is a choice and it's yours, rather than *having* to do something because you are at the effect of something or someone else.

- ➤ I *want* to eat salad for lunch
- ➤ I *want* to cook healthily for dinner tonight
- ➤ I *want* to go for a 5 mile run

It sounds a lot different from *having* to do those things doesn't it? Just have a go at this to get a feel for how it changes your interpretation of the proposed activity.

Another word that is so small yet becomes so important in your vocabulary is the word 'try'. We hear it all the time, and whilst we don't notice the real meaning consciously, we definitely do unconsciously. 'Try' implies a lot of effort with no results. Imagine this scenario; you are a manager at work and you ask one of your team to produce a report for you and give it to you by 4pm tomorrow. They respond and say: "yes, sure, I'll *try* and get that to you tomorrow for 4pm." We all know that chances are that it's never going to happen. How many times have you *tried* to lose weight? How many times have you *tried* to eat well, or *tried* to stop eating junk food?

Let's do a little experiment together. If you are sitting down reading this then *try* and stand up, and if you're already standing then *try* and sit down.

How did you get on?

Did you manage to stand if you were sitting? *Really?* I asked you to *try* and stand up, not to *stand* up.

Do it again. *Try* and stand up. I bet you are straining while you're sitting there motioning to get up. In reality you are still sitting there (or vice versa). You see, you're either standing up or sitting down – you can't *try* to do either. Need further proof? If there's a chair near you *try* and pick it up. Can you? No. You're either picking up the chair or not picking up the chair. It's like a binary sequence, 0 or 1, on or off.

Perhaps you saw the second Star Wars movie when you were growing up, or perhaps even as an adult? It's called *'The Empire Strikes Back'*. Anyway, there's a great scene in it with the Master Jedi trainer, Yoda, and his apprentice, Luke Skywalker. Luke is undergoing his training and is practising mastering his skills in using 'The Force' to pick up rocks with his mind when suddenly his spaceship sinks into a swamp. Luke doesn't believe they can get it out of there and Yoda then teaches Luke a valuable lesson.

LUKE: "Oh, no. We'll never get it out now."

YODA: "So certain are you. Always with you it *cannot* be done. Hear you nothing that I say?"

LUKE: "Master, moving stones around is one thing. This is totally different."

YODA: "No! No different! **Only different in your mind**. You must unlearn what you have learned."

LUKE: "All right, I'll give it a *try*."

YODA: "No! *Try* not. **Do. Or do not**. There is no *try*."

There is so much in that small passage about beliefs and conditioning on what we think. In particular, the last line illustrates the point I'm making. *"Do. Or do not. There is no try."* You either do something or you don't do something - either way you can't *'try'* and do it. Now that I've raised your awareness to the word *try*, I guarantee that you'll hear it all the time and be especially tuned to it when you hear someone say that they'll *try* and get something done.

When I used to work in the Financial Services industry, I worked for a very skilled boss and he was especially good at picking up when people said in a meeting that they would *try* and do something. He wouldn't let them leave until they'd verbally spoken the commitment to getting it done. He wanted to hear them say: "I will get this done by xxxx time." Not just: "I'll try and get it done" or agreeing once he'd picked up on the word 'try'. You had to say the commitment back to him out loud. And I've got to say that it works. Once you say the whole thing out loud, it's like something gets registered in your unconscious and because you've made this commitment out loud you find it almost impossible to break.

How else does language affect what you will do and your progress towards your goals? I touched on it earlier with beliefs but using words like "I can't" does not serve you. If you think you can, or you think you can't, you're right, remember? What if you truly can't do something? It might be true to say that you can't run 10 miles, but how could you re-phrase that to better serve you? Here are some ideas:

"I can't run ten miles, **yet.**"

"I'm **working towards** running ten miles."

"I'm **in training** to run ten miles."

"I'm **building up** my endurance to **be able to** run ten miles."

All statements convey the message that you are currently not able to complete ten miles, but internally, to your unconscious mind, you are instructing it that you will be able to do so in the future. These statements pre-suppose that you will be able to run 10 miles *some day*. If you say you can't do something, your brain will go off to think of all the reasons why that's true. If you say to yourself (and others) that you are working towards something, your brain will go off and search for ways in which to meet that objective. It will do all this unconsciously and it won't take any effort on your part. As long as your brain works for you in this way, isn't it better to get it working *for* you and your goals, rather than against?

Here's something else now for you to consider. When you talk about your goals for health, weight loss and fitness state them in the positive and make them positive goals. Rather than say "I want to lose weight" (which is talking about what you don't want – i.e. the weight) say what you *do* want – "I want to be fit, healthy and full of vitality". Also be specific in your outcome as 'lose weight' is so generic. Every time you go to the toilet you 'lose weight'. Your unconscious mind feels like it's succeeded as you've met your goal! Have a *specific* weight range in mind. I recommend a weight range as you will almost never be exactly the weight that you want and your unconscious mind is quite literal, so if you say that you want to be 10 stone, it will think 10 stone exactly, not 9 stone 12 and not 10 stone 2 - but 10 stone exactly. Better to have a weight range of something manageable like between 9 stone 10 and 10 stone 4 (in kilograms that's roughly 62 kg to 65 kg). It's important to have the range as you will always fluctuate in weight – even weighing yourself in the same place and with the same clothes or food in your stomach. When you have a range and you notice that you're going too far to either extreme of the range, you can then take corrective measures.

Another reason why you should drop the word 'lose' is because anything that the body sees as a loss it will fight to retain. Nobody really likes losing anything, do they? Think about it for a second, would you work harder to *earn* a thousand pounds or to stop someone from *stealing* a thousand pounds?

In 2004, I learnt firsthand about how you always move in the direction of what you focus on. I was snowboarding in Austria and heading towards a jump when I noticed I was going faster than I was comfortable with, so I started to slow down. This altered my trajectory slightly and I moved off my approach line. As this happened I noticed a little tree stump near to where the jump was and as I focussed on the tree stump, instead of the take off point, I moved towards it and BAM! I hit it full force. This resulted in a serious shoulder injury and about 12 months of physiotherapy; but the point is this. Because I was focussing on what I didn't want, I ended up getting just that! When all I needed to do was focus on where I wanted to go. The same is true of the saying 'lose weight'. Saying that you want to *lose weight* is focussing on what you want to avoid – the weight.

Language is one of the primary ways of how we communicate to each other and ourselves and by changing the way that we describe events we can directly change the experience and therefore the emotion that we attach to that experience. By way of example, if I were to miss a bus which meant I was going to be a few minutes late for a meeting I might say all manner of things to myself (or out loud) like:

"Stupid Hari, why didn't I leave earlier?"

"Oh ****, I'm going to be ******* late now!"

How about if you changed some of those words?

"Silly Hari, why didn't I leave earlier?"

"Darn it, I'm going to be a wee bit late now."

Does that *feel* differently to you? The words that we choose to describe our experiences *become* our experiences and so we need to choose them wisely. There are estimated to be somewhere between 1 – 2 million words in the English language (depending on whether you include words from botany, chemistry, slang, dialects etc). Although the average person might be familiar (from a sample of 100,000) with about 50% of them; in the average person's active vocabulary, the number of words regularly used is closer to only 2000. The bible uses 8000 words and Shakespeare used 24,000 – even inventing some himself. Furthermore, there are approximately 4000 words to describe emotional states but amazingly 3600 of these describe negative experiences. It's no wonder that people find it a lot easier to describe their emotions in a negative way than a positive way. Take a minute now to write down all the emotions you feel on a day-to-day basis. Just think over the last week and write them down in the space below or in your notebook.

Emotions Identification Process

Emotions I've experienced on a day-to-day basis in the last week are:

_____ _____ _____ _____

_____ _____ _____ _____

_____ _____ _____ _____

_____ _____ _____ _____

_____ _____ _____ _____

_____ _____ _____

I'm betting that the majority of you wrote between 8 – 12 words and that around 75% of those were negative. I've done this process myself and also been in a room with over a thousand other people and that was the average. It's astonishing really considering there are 400 positive emotions to choose from and we might only be experiencing three or four of them on a day-to-day basis.

I hope that this process has illustrated just how we use our language and how it changes how we **re**present our experiences by the words that we use to describe them. By changing our vocabulary, it will change what we choose to make our reality and therefore what we can achieve. Spend some time over the next week making a conscious effort to work on the advice given above and notice the change in your outlook to activities and also your **re**presentation of your experiences.

Chapter Summary

- ✓ The words we use to describe our experiences actually become our experiences. What and how we say it is integral to how we feel about an activity or experience
- ✓ By changing the words we use it will change how we feel about an experience.
- ✓ There are several times more words to describe negative emotional states than there are words to describe positive ones.
- ✓ You wrote down all the emotions you have felt on a day-to-day basis over the last week.

7 - Food

I'm Greek and for Greeks, food is a major part of our culture. I've never really been a smoker, nor have I ever been a massive drinker. But, if ever there were one weakness for me, it would be food. I love it. As a kid, I was quite a fussy eater - some would say I'm worse now! My favourite foods as a toddler were ice cream, bread and butter. I was also a meat and potatoes fan who would occasionally eat a bit of cucumber. I was the kind of person that would eat (no word of lie) 18 roast potatoes in a single sitting! Just ask my sisters. When I was 16, I started eating some salad along with meat and potatoes, but only if there were any gaps on the plate which were not already occupied by the meat and potatoes! It wasn't until I went to university at 19 that I started to eat vegetables regularly. And you want to know why? It was only because I was in a catered hall and we used to get only two to four potatoes with our evening meal. I could never survive on that! I had no choice but to eat vegetables unless I wanted to feel hungry. Still – even with eating my vegetables it didn't prevent me from jumping the fence about two hours later to go to the local kebab shop. I can't believe it now, but I used to buy donner kebabs all the time. For those of you that don't already know, a donner kebab is the worst kind of kebab you can get – it's the lowest quality meat from the spit that rotates all day long. In fact, I used to eat an average of four a week. I ate so many that I even got a free T-shirt from the owner. You had to have eaten 50 kebabs to get to that level!

What's the point in me telling you all this? Well, just like you perhaps, I know what it's like to be at the mercy of food. Junk food was my vice - be it the dirty donner kebabs, a Burger King, KFC, McDonald's, those little breaded Chicken Kiev's, Sara Lee's chocolate gateaux, Ferrero Rocher chocolates or M&M's... the list goes on. Eating incorrectly is obviously the largest contributing factor to excess weight and you may or may not know that eating the wrong things (and plenty of them) is also the cause of many other of life's ailments: indigestion, heartburn, constipation, diarrhoea, headaches, kidney stones, type-2 diabetes, gout and nausea. These can all be traced back to the quality of your diet. What you put into your body is primarily required as fuel. The quality of the food you put in will determine the quality in performance you get from it. Rubbish in, rubbish out. Good stuff in, good stuff out. It's as simple as that. I mean you wouldn't spend lots of money to attain an amazing sports car and fill it with budget poor quality oil and diesel when it needs petrol, would you?

The secret to shedding the pounds isn't really a secret at all – it's to eat less and exercise more. That's it in a nutshell. Obviously that's a bit of an oversimplification and there are other considerations which may play a play, but essentially that's it. It's so simple and obvious that people often look at *anything* but the obvious.

It's *emotional* eating which tends to leave people into the wrong place physically. When you have a physical necessity to eat, it's more of a gradual build up of hunger, while emotional eating is more to do with *having* to have it right then and there – there's a sense of urgency about it. Sometimes, the emotional side is just to make you feel good or perhaps you're having a great dinner with someone and you don't want the evening to end. Maybe eating that cake reminds you of being a child at your grandparent's home and that makes you feel happy. Either way, it's an emotional trigger that's prompting the action to eat more. How can we stop this from happening? The first step is to have an awareness of the action, which you already have achieved now that you're reading all this. Once you become aware of this habit of emotional eating, it will make you more finely tuned to realising when this happens in the future. So once you realise that you're eating a particular cake, not because you need it, but because it provides you with some kind of emotional attachment to your grandparent's house, you regain power over the action. But is there a way to get that feeling you want *without* eating the food?

There are a few techniques to do this and the process I'm going to give here is just one of these. It's called anchoring. It's a way to associate a feeling to an action, object, expression or anything else. It's something we've all been doing for years, whether we realised it or not. Advertisers know it and have used it to great effect for decades. Have you ever heard a piece of music that reminds you of a certain holiday, or time in your past? Have you ever smelled someone's perfume and which reminded you of a past relationship or present love? Have you ever walked past the golden arches of McDonalds and stepped inside even though you weren't really hungry? This is anchoring. You see, what happens is that through repeated exposure to some kind of trigger (sound, smell, touch, visual cue etc) while in a heightened emotional state, that trigger (provided it is unique to you) will literally 'anchor' (like a ships anchor) the feeling that you hold at that time, to that trigger.

That's why you might find yourself smiling (or sad) when you smell that perfume. Or why you might get all energised hearing a piece of music that you loved as a 17 year old while on summer holiday. These are all accidental anchors; created unconsciously, if you like. In that you weren't aware at the time that you were making them, but you have them all the same. What we'll do here is take you through a process to create anchors consciously for your use in a positive way.

Think of the emotional state that you would like. If, for example, you tend to eat when you are stressed and you think that eating calms you down, then I want you to think of three examples of when you were calm. Or if you can't think of one, then think about someone else who you know is able to remain calm. It might not be calmness for you – you might eat when you don't need to (for example at some networking function) because you need to feel confident or sociable with company.

Anchoring Process

Start by completing the following statement about when you overeat:

I tend to overeat (or eat the wrong food) when I'm

_____

(anxious, stressed, bored, shy, lonely, hurt etc)

Now, think of something that you want to have in place of that, so if you eat because in social situations you are shy, then perhaps you want to feel more sociable naturally. I'll use the example of shy/sociable below, but you choose what you want. Read the entire exercise first and then do it. Alternatively find someone who can walk you through it so you can focus on the exercise rather than reading it and doing it at the same time. Go to http://thethoughtgym.com/book for guided support.

1. Think of a time in your past when you had this positive state (e.g. sociability).

2. As you think of that time, really get back to being there. See what you saw, feel what you felt, hear what you heard and smell what you smelled. Really live it, be there again, and as you get close to the peak of that emotion, squeeze your left thumb and little finger tightly together. This is called 'anchoring' and to get back to the state again all you have to do is do the same unique action again (in this case squeezing your left thumb and little finger together).

3. After 5-15 seconds of holding your thumb and little finger together release them.

4. Now break state. What's your favourite TV show?

5. Think of a second example for when you felt really (sociable).

6. As you think of that time, really get back to being there. See what you saw, feel what you felt, hear what you heard and smell what you smelled. Really live it, be there again, and as you get close to the peak of that emotion, squeeze your left thumb and little finger tightly together. (Here we're building upon this trigger.)

7. Really feel that emotion of (sociability) as you squeeze your left thumb and little finger together. Intensify your feeling of (sociability) by 50%, 100%, 1000%!

8. After 5-15 seconds of holding your thumb and little finger together release.

9. Now break state. What was last thing you bought at the shops?

10. Think of a third example for when you felt really (sociable).

11. As you think of that time, really get back to being there. See what you saw, feel what you felt, hear what you heard and smell what you smelled. Really live it, be there again, and as you get close to the peak of that emotion, squeeze your left thumb and little finger tightly together.

12. Really feel that emotion of (sociability) as you squeeze your left thumb and little finger together. Intensify your feeling of (sociability) by 50%, 100%, 1000%!

13. After 5-15 seconds of holding your thumb and little finger together release.

14. Now break state. What posters did you have in your room as a child?

What happens now when you squeeze your thumb and little finger together? What do you feel? If it's not strong enough go back to that (sociable) state and repeat the process. I find with this one that the challenge sometimes lies in really getting back into that state again in your mind. So now that you know how to create an 'anchor' I suggest that you use the same trigger again when you really *are* in that state for real and 'anchor' to it. It will build on the anchor and make it work with increasing intensity. Here we used a physical trigger of our thumb and little finger but you can use any physical movement you want as a trigger – or even a word or action - to get you back to your desired state.

The next time that you find yourself in a situation where you are reaching for the buffet table to feel more (sociable), fire off your trigger and rely on that instead and not the food to satisfy your emotional craving.

So, if it's that simple and obvious why is there such a problem in Western society with obesity? Why is it that you picked up this book? Is there a way to eat what you want and get slimmer? The answer to the last question is yes – kind of! Sorry to be so non-committal but I don't want people to walk away from reading this book thinking they can eat whatever they want and be healthy. There is a way to eat some of what you want and be healthier and I will give you some information in this chapter which will definitely help with that but I won't pretend that this is all I would advocate. I'll also give you information to help you make better food choices in the first place. Just imagine finding out that you actually start to *want* different types of food – that would be good, wouldn't it?

What I *would* advocate though would be to eat as many foods which are high in nutrients and minerals. These are the vital constituents of food that your body can really get fuel from. Things like green leafy vegetables, other fresh vegetables and whole grains are essential – interestingly, they are foods close to their natural state and not altered by man. Any foods like that are best for you.

I'm not a dietician so what I'm going to do is share with you my personal story, research and knowledge about diet. As I mentioned already, I used to be a huge meat eater. In fact, I ate it twice a day without fail. But that changed a while ago. Each year for lent I give something up for a few weeks. I'm not religious, but I find it's a good time of year to give up something (or start something – if it's something that's good for you!) as it's a finite stretch of time. This also makes it easy to explain your actions to friends without receiving resistance and so it becomes more achievable. In the past I have given up alcohol, bread, television and even meat once before too! So when I decided to give up meat this time, I knew I should be able to do it.

This time however, it was remarkably easier to give up meat than back when I last did it in 2002. And when I did eat a bit of meat on Easter Sunday - I felt terrible. I was wiped out, felt lethargic, sick and needed to sleep straight away. What I then also realised was that throughout lent I had felt more energised, needed less sleep and better still - I could eat more. My theory was that without the burden of having to digest any meat, my body didn't need to use up valuable time and energy resources when I went to sleep, and so it was able to rest and repair itself more efficiently.

I later found out that there is a theory about how the biggest drain on the body's energy resources is actually the act of digestion itself. This was popularised in the book 'Fit for Life' by Harvey and Marilyn Diamond. The Diamonds then also went on to describe a process known as 'food combining' which they claimed was necessary in order to get the best return on energy expenditure for food consumed.

'Food combining' is really about what types of food you can and can't eat together – mainly because of how they are digested in the body. When proteins are eaten, your body secretes acids to break them down. When you eat starches, your body secretes alkali to break that down. But when you eat them both together e.g. meat and potatoes; your body secretes both acid and alkali – each neutralising the other and your food then fails to digest properly as the body starts secreting even more acids and alkali in an attempt to digest the food. This is all still a bit controversial but in a way, and based on my own experiences, it makes sense to me – certainly the bit about digestion being a big consumer of energy. I mean, have you ever eaten so much at dinner that you struggled to get to sleep? I know I have. True, we don't do this daily (I hope!), but the times when it does happen, just accentuates what happens anyway with normal quantities.

Now however, because I still currently don't eat meat, even if I do overeat at dinner, I find that I digest the food I've eaten much quicker. A fact I attribute to the meal not consisting of meat and hence, by default, I'm combining my foods well, as the Diamond's suggest doing. Also, because it takes more effort to digest meat than it does vegetables, then it also makes sense to me that if I don't eat meat then I make the best use of my sleep. This is because I am able to allow the body to focus on recovery and repair rather than digestion. This is true even if I were to combine food the right way i.e. meat and vegetables only with no starches.

There is a lot of information already out there highlighting current popular opinion relating to meat and how much or what type to eat so I won't be going into all that in this book. But just by way of example, in March 2012 the results of a 30-year Harvard Medical School study confirmed that diets consisting of red meat led to increased risks of death, cancer and heart disease. Like I said, I was a big meat eater – you would be hard pushed to find a more dedicated meat eater than me. I thought – in fact I had a belief so strong – that I could *never* survive long term without meat. My belief has, of course, changed now, based on learning new information and expanding my awareness on such issues. The information below is given in the spirit that, by knowing a bit more, you will be able to make more informed decisions about your food choices and what fuels your body. My goal with the next few pages is not to make you a vegetarian or vegan, but to show you that there's nothing to be afraid of should you make the choice to re-examine how much meat you eat.

The first thing that I usually get asked when I tell people that I don't eat meat is "but where do you get your protein from?" Well, in actual fact I still eat fish, (although maybe that will change in the future). Assuming that I don't eat fish either, then where would I get my protein from? First of all, how much protein does the human body actually need? Not all authorities agree on how much protein your body requires with estimates continually changing over time. Figures from the American Journal of Clinical Nutrition give a low end of 2.5 % of your daily calorific intake to be from protein. The World Health Organisation figures vary depending on what paper you read and can range from 4.5 % to 10%, and the National Research Council refers to a figure of about 10%. Generally though, most reports mention about 0.8g per kg of lean muscle mass per day. So for a 75kg man this equates to about 60g of protein. There are 4 calories in each gram of protein, so that equals to 240 calories. Less than 10% of the 2500 calories per day recommended allowance. Of course, I've also read other articles, particularly to do with body-building, which quote much higher figures – up to 30% of your daily calorific intake, in some cases. Let common sense be your guide though and consider this first. At what stage of your life do you think you need to grow the most and thus need the most protein for growth? I propose that it's when we (literally) were making noticeable and weekly size changes – when we were babies, yes? The growth that's experienced at that stage of life is massive compared to anything we experience later, and the average baby would only be getting their nutrition from their own mother's milk – and guess how much protein is in mother's milk? It's between 1.6% and 4%. And that's what we need at a time when we really need to grow.

What if we need to get 10% of our calories from protein – the higher end of the scale, well - just take a look at the protein content of some vegetables, legumes and fruits to get an idea of what protein levels they provide, as a percentage of calories they contain.

Legumes	Protein Percentage	Nuts and Seeds	Protein Percentage
Soybean sprouts	54%	Pumpkin Seeds	21%
Tofu	43%	Sunflower Seeds	17%
Soybean	35%	Almonds	12%
Lentils	29%	Cashews	12%
Vegetables		**Vegetables**	
Spinach	49%	Parsley	34%
Watercress	46%	Lettuce	34%
Kale	45%	Zucchini	26%
Broccoli	45%	Cucumber	24%
Brussels Sprouts	44%	Celery	21%
Cauliflower	40%	Potato	11%

But isn't there such a thing as good protein sources like those only coming from meat and dairy? The incredibly well researched book, *A Diet for a New America*, by John Robbins gives a good explanation on about proteins and this misconception about good and bad proteins, so is worth reading, but I'll summarise the key points here. The idea that animal proteins are superior appeared in a study from 1914 when two researchers, Osborne and Mendel, performed laboratory tests on rats and found that the rats developed faster with animal protein than plant protein. It was after that, that this idea of class A and class B protein quality entered the public consciousness.

The issue was further muddled in the 1940's with further studies showing that certain amino acids (our body's building blocks) when removed from a rats diet, harmed its growth. Various experiments later and scientists discovered that a specific combination of amino acids produced the best growth. It was a pattern that was similar to that found in eggs. The egg then became the gold standard for protein comparison.

Later, in the 1960's the notion was popularised that the body could get all its essential amino acids - mixed together in a way akin to that of an egg - from vegetables. That was, if you combined the vegetables properly (the body needs 20 amino acids and 11 of these are produced by the body anyway - the other 9 being the 'essential' ones). This was due in a large part to a lady called Frances Moore Lappe who promoted this idea in her book, *Diet for a Small Planet*. When properly combined, the proteins in vegetables matched or exceeded those in eggs and meat.

Unfortunately, this 'gold standard' of the egg being the best example of a complete protein source was based on a study done on rats – something that Lappe didn't know at the time. In the following years Lappe published revised editions of her book where she emphasised that the inference that she made in the original book - that in order for the body to use protein effectively it needed to resemble that of an animal protein - was misleading and that with a healthy and varied diet, protein combining is not necessary.

When populations around the world are studied, statistics consistently show that those populations with vegetarian or near vegetarian diets live longer, have better health and are more active than their Western counterparts. Even Arnold Schwarzenegger says that for "basic good eating: eat one gram of protein for every two pounds of body weight" – which would be way less than the amount some diets recommend which is 30%, 40% or even more.

I also hear the argument about iron deficiency. The reality is though, that per 100 calories, spinach has 11 milligrams (mg) of iron, cucumber 7 mg but sirloin steak about 1.9 mg, and chicken breast 0.8 mg. And there's a lot of iron in other vegetables too so you shouldn't fall short of iron provided that you're getting a good balance of fresh vegetables in your diet.

I was concerned that, even knowing all the information above, that because I'm quite active, I wouldn't have the endurance for anything if I stopped eating meat. Maybe you're thinking the same thing? Especially as after reading this book you will no doubt want to exercise more. Interestingly enough for me though, in the course of my research, I read about Professor Irving Fisher of Yale University who studied three groups of volunteers. The groups were meat eating athletes, vegetarian athletes and vegetarian sedentary people. Fisher found that the vegetarian athletes performed best out of the group, followed by the vegetarian sedentary people when it came to endurance. Subsequent studies have also lent credence to this idea.

And just to illustrate and debunk the idea that if you're vegetarian you aren't able to perform as well athletically; here are some people who have accomplished some extraordinary feats.

> Bill Pearl: Four time Mr Universe bodybuilding champion.
> Martina Navratilova: Tennis player with 18 Grand Slam victories and one of the best female tennis players of the 20th century.

> ➢ Robert Parish: Legendary basketball player inducted into the NBA Hall of Fame.
> ➢ Dave Scott: Holds the record of the most Ironman Triathlon victories. (An Ironman triathlon is a 2.4 mile swim, 112 miles cycle followed by a marathon.)
> ➢ Carl Lewis: Adopted a vegan diet ahead of 1991 World Athletics Championships and ran the race of his life. Often cited as being the greatest ever Olympian.
> ➢ Edwin Moses: Olympic Gold medallist who went 8 years without losing in the 400 metre hurdles in the 1970's and 1980's.

All of them had vegetarian diets. And guess what other vegetarians are out there that seem to me to be pretty strong? Gorillas; and what about elephants, rhinoceroses, hippos and buffalos? They all seem to do just fine without eating meat. Additionally, vegetarian animals, like the orang-utan, only need about 6 hours of sleep a day and a giraffe about 2 hours. How many hours does a lion need? 20 hours a day. I could go on, as there are countless examples but the point that I'm making is this. Should you choose it, you don't *need* meat to be fit and healthy. Provided that you have a varied diet, full of (or as close as possible to) natural and unprocessed foods from a wide selection of sources, you will be OK.

In comparison to vegetable and plant sources, meat is high in fat and low in water content – completely in contradiction to what the human body actually needs. As humans, we don't have enough of the enzymes we need to digest the meat properly anyway. The fact that we are considered (by many) to be omnivores and can eat anything (although there are many who actually say that we are really herbivores by design); it shouldn't detract from the fact that we are not out and out carnivores, designed to eat meat. Our intestine tract is long and windy and designed for the slow absorption of plant based food. It's not short and direct like that of a lion which is designed to pass rapidly decaying meat out of its system quickly.

This isn't a nutrition book, so I recommend you read more and also perhaps consult a registered professional. But just bear in mind the following before taking advice from anyone; what's their motivation, what's their professional and personal experience, what do opposing views argue and what has been scientifically proven and who funded that research? Was it the government, big business, the meat or dairy industry? Just know where you're getting your information from and make informed decisions, is all I ask. Test it and see if it works for you. Don't blindly believe what I (or anyone else) has to say, but do use it as a guide. I give my personal experiences and there will be differing opinions from others. Just remember that if you're currently in a place where something has to change, and what you've been doing up to now hasn't been working, I suggest that you must do something – *any*thing – else. Do something different. There's no point doing the same thing over and over again and expecting different results.

When you're in danger, you're probably aware that your body releases adrenaline via the 'fight or flight' response. Like it does in humans, the same thing happens with animals. So let me ask you a question now. Do you think that when an animal is about to be slaughtered it senses that they're about to get killed? You bet they do – whatever any meat lover might tell you. It knows all right and that causes it to stimulate its 'fight or flight' response and release a lot of adrenaline into its body – just at the moment it's killed. And where does all that adrenaline go? It remains in the meat for happy digestion by us. I think that it's now widely accepted that a child's diet can dramatically affect their behaviour.

Take them off all the sodas, chocolates and other processed and refined foods and their behaviour has been shown to improve. Just watch Morgan Spurlock's documentary, *SuperSize Me,* to see one example of a school which improved the student's behaviour just by improving the menu. So let's extend that thinking further. If such obvious examples (soda, sugars etc) affect children's behaviours, is it such a leap to think that eating products laced with adrenaline from an animal's 'fight or flight' response might affect *our* behaviour in some way? It's my personal view, but I don't think that I'm alone in this.

> *"The time will come when men such as me will look on the murder of animals as they now look on the murder of men" – Leonard da Vinci*

> *"As long as there are slaughterhouses, there will be battlefields."*
> *- Leo Tolstoy*

I think that most of us would agree that both Leonardo da Vinci and Leo Tolstoy knew a thing or two. And you know what; they weren't the only vegetarians to have accomplished something worthwhile and left their mark on humanity. What about Einstein, Thomas Edison, Voltaire, Isaac Newton, Gandhi, Abraham Lincoln, Plato, Pythagoras and Socrates? A search on Google will give you a few more. My personal experience is that since going meat-free, I have had a lot more focus, greater clarity of thought and calmness with better sleep, more energy and better attention. Perhaps the meat-free diet helped those 'greats' achieve all they did – if so, I hope I'm on the right path. I would be happy if, by writing this book, I can influence you to just investigate matters further and you might just find that that is the one thing that makes the difference for you and helps you lead a healthier lifestyle. If I accomplish that, then the effort in writing this book would have been worth it. All I can say is that up to now I have found being meat-free great for me. And the same can be said of dairy.

I stopped eating dairy in 2008 after finally deciding to trial it for lent. I had heard that dairy consumption might be the reason for my sinus issues, and also by reducing or eliminating dairy it might also help the tinnitus I had. Another great motivation point for me was that at that time chocolate was a big part of my work colleagues' daily ritual and I knew that was just going to be trouble for me. In my experience, people don't *really* appreciate the big picture of decisions they make, such as eating a bit of extra chocolate - but it all adds up. A Mars bar a day (to help you work, rest and play!) has 230 calories and 12g of fat and equates to an extra 3kg of fat for you each year. Do you fancy gaining half a stone a year just because of your 3pm munchies?

Again, for me, trialling abstinence from dairy for lent worked; as I could always see an end point that I could 'quit' the regime and go back to eating dairy. What I found though, was that I felt better, my sinuses improved, my tinnitus improved and what's more, I didn't have as much gas! And you know what, it was quite easy. Sure, in the beginning switching to soya milk felt weird, but after a couple of weeks I got used to it – in fact, the cells in our taste buds last for only around 10 days so abstaining from something for a period of time greater than this and you will start to lose the 'taste' for it. Now it feels weird and even sickly if I have normal milk. I mix up soya milk these days with oat, rice, hemp, coconut or almond milk for variety because sticking to one food type day after day isn't great for you – variety is the spice of life after all! And there are other 'margarines' that you could use instead such as soya or olive oil – you would never tell the difference. You can even get vegan soft cream cheese (just like 'Philadelphia' spread) such as the brand Sheese, which tastes even better! There are so many dairy free options these days that it's easy to make the switch once you realise that there *are* alternatives. But why make the switch in the first place, you may well ask? And where would you get your calcium from?

Well the answer isn't to eat dairy. I'll get back to the calcium question in a moment, but let me just mention that excessive dairy intake also blocks the absorption of iron into the system. So if you give up meat only to substitute it with dairy, then you're running the risk of not getting enough iron because a) as mentioned, dairy blocks iron absorption and b) you're probably crowding out a lot of the other food groups like grains and vegetables that would add to your iron intake. Many of the adult population in the West are lactose intolerant – some sources estimate it to be as high as 30%, although the NHS gives a more modest figure of 5% (of UK adults) to be lactose intolerant. For other ethnicities, however, for example Hispanic, South Indian or black this is 50%-80% and for American Indians and Asians it's almost 100%. Lactose intolerance can occur at different times but for most Caucasians, it usually affects children above the age of four but for other ethnicities it's as early as two. Most mammals normally become lactose intolerant after their weaning months/years. This is because they are not able to produce the enzyme lactase, which is needed for successful digestion of lactose, the sugar found in milk.

Nowadays you can buy lacto-free milk but it's still from cow's milk and not great for you as I'll cover shortly. Do you not think that it's strange that out of all the species on earth, we're the only ones that still consume milk past infancy? And not even milk from our own species. Doesn't that give you a clue as to whether we should be consuming it or not?

So let's get back to the calcium question and where to get it from. All leafy green vegetables are inherently high in calcium (and a bunch of other good stuff for you like iron, Vitamin C and the rest) as are things like celery, cauliflower, onions, tofu, green beans, almonds and more still. Provided that you're eating a varied diet with lots of varied vegetables and getting the calories you need, then you will be getting enough calcium. And if you think that vegetables are boring (as I once did) then you just need to experiment with using different herbs and spices or simply a bit of lemon. A quick vegetable stir-fry is easy, versatile and tasty as is just some steamed vegetables with a bit of flaxseed oil and lemon drizzled over the top.

Why else wouldn't you want to consume dairy? Well, for one, it's believed by many (including me in my experience) to be very mucus forming. It's true that having some mucus does play an important role in keeping us safe from toxins that we allow to enter our bodies, but too much not only gives bad sinuses but also promotes the growth of negative microforms. These are essentially yeasts, fungus, mould, bacteria and viruses – all nasty stuff. Their toxic wastes can produce many troubling symptoms in the body. Too much mucus can also lead to poor digestion, lung congestion and constant throat clearing. Also, like many animal products, dairy products contain all sorts of nice hormone and pesticide residues as well as other microforms which do you no good – not to mention all that saturated fat. Dairy is also very acid-forming within your body and while I'm not going to go into this here, the basic idea is that you want your body to be very slightly alkali (your blood should retain a pH balance of about 7.365). As it takes about 20 parts of alkali to neutralise one part of acid, the basic premise is acid=bad and alkali=good when it comes to what you put in your body and the reaction that food has on your body.

Now that the issue around food has been lightly touched on, I want to give you some tips, advice and information about food which is unrelated to the kind of diet you eat and which, I hope, will be easy and effortless for you to consider and implement. In addition to what you eat, equally as important for weight maintenance is *how* you eat.

According to figures from the World Health Organisation in 2005, about 1.6 billion people are overweight – the figure for those in the UK is over 60% and in the US over 70%. So why are so many people overweight? Put simply, eating too much and of the wrong types of food and not exercising enough. Why do we overeat? Usually eating when you're not *truly* hungry comes down to some description of emotional eating. How many times have you reached for food because you were bored, stressed, lonely, hurt, sad or even being entertained – like watching a movie or a show? It doesn't help that we're part of a society brainwashed and encouraged to eat whenever we can. You go to the cinema and there's all manner of temptations; you go for a loo break at work and you pass the vending machine filled with crisps and chocolates. Temptation is all around us. It's on billboards, on TV and online. Adverts are designed to make us think that a certain product will mean something to us – some kind of pleasurable experience for us. Need a break? Have a Kit-Kat. Want it your way? Grab a Burger King. Want a feeling of 'lovin it'? Try the golden arches at McDonald's. And the problem isn't in just eating when we don't need to but how often have you finished your plate even when you *weren't* hungry? I know I have – all the time.

We've been conditioned since birth to finish our food – "Think about those starving kids in Africa" - your parents used to say when you didn't want to finish your meal. I used to be terrible with this, especially being brought up in a Greek family where if I didn't have at least three servings my parents feared that I might waste away! And I have to say that overeating is probably one of the biggest challenges I'm faced with when it came to my health and weight. I do exercise a lot, and that definitely helps. It increases your metabolic rate as well as actually burning the fuel through the exercise itself – but even so, as you age, natural changes occur and so I wouldn't dream that today I could put into my body what I did 10 or 20 years ago and still look and feel like I do now. It's just not possible. But I like to cook – and often it's for one. I never cook for one though. Usually it will be for four. Two portions for dinner and then two for lunch! If I made something particularly appealing – in my meat-eating days it might be a carbonara with bacon for example (albeit a low fat dairy-free version. I substitute the bacon for grilled aubergine instead now.) I could easily find myself eating the whole lot in one sitting. And then not being able to move! One tactic that I use when I feel that a meal might be so nice I would want to eat the lot, is before I even sit down at the table, I pack the lunch portion away in the container I'll be taking with me and put it out of sight. Once it's gone, my brain automatically thinks it's eating all that is available to it. It works for me, and I think it will work for you too.

It takes about 20 minutes for your brain to catch up with your stomach once you've eaten something so although you may *think* that you're hungry, you might in fact not be. Here are some tips that are *so* easy to implement and will literally help you maintain a good weight and ensure that you eat just what you need. Experiment with them for the next 30 days and notice the difference.

Chew food slowly – Food starts to break down in your mouth, not your stomach and by chewing food slower and for a longer period of time it will release enzymes in your mouth which help to digest the food and break it down even before it hits the stomach. Just chew for 25% longer than you normally do.

Focus *only* on eating – Don't be distracted by watching TV or reading or making phone calls or doing any other kind of multi-tasking. Studies show that you eat more when occupied doing other activities. Multi-tasking doesn't work – our brains are much like computers which can really only do one thing at a time – computers just happen to do it really quickly and then move on to next thing. It's also said in Buddhist philosophy that if you do more than one thing at a time, you actually do nothing at all, so take time to enjoy your meals properly and give mealtime the necessary focus.

Enjoy each mouthful – A lot of people lead busy lives and although they might constantly think about food all day, when it comes to eating it, instead of enjoying every bite, they just wolf it down. Make sure that when you finally get to eat, you take your time and enjoy the process of eating. Practice the art of 'mindfulness' and be conscious of your eating – *even* if you're eating a Mars bar. Focus on each bite as you take it. Can you still manage to finish it?

Save the leftovers – Before you sit down to eat, save any leftovers (don't leave them easily accessible) and only put on your plate what you think you really need to satisfy your hunger. You should walk away from the table feeling satisfied, not crawl away feeling stuffed. If you're in a restaurant then ask for a 'doggy bag' at the beginning of the meal, rather than at the end or not at all. Most of us feel compelled to finish everything that's put in front of us – especially if we've paid for it.

Drink a large glass of water – Rather than snacking just before food - drink a large glass of water. The fullness in your stomach will often ease the hunger pangs until you can cook something healthy. Most of the time it's dehydration that is mistaken by the brain for hunger (the brain is 85% water) and so drinking water should always be your first point of call when feeling hungry.

When you're full, stop – If you find it a challenge to leave something on your plate; then start by leaving just *something*, anything really. Even if it's only a single chip or mouthful of rice! It will start to send the right messages to your brain that you are able to leave food on the plate and that it's OK. Continuing to eat when you don't need it means the body can't burn it. It is like filling a car full of petrol every week when you only drive 20 miles a week. Pretty soon it will start to spill out the sides – much like those love handles.

Eat when you want to – If you starve yourself, your body's starvation mode will start to set in and slow your metabolism down to conserve energy. Do it often enough, and you'll begin to store food whenever you eat it instead of burning it for fuel. I'm never particularly mindful of what time it is, I'll eat whenever I'm hungry.

Labels everywhere – Start to use labels on your food cabinets or fridge. Put a big question mark on your fridge – that will break your pattern from just unconsciously reaching for the food when you're not really hungry. Often, if we just consciously act rather than unconsciously react, we make different choices. You could even tape some Post-It's® to your cookie jar or sweet cupboard, with questions like "are you really sure you need this?" Or "are you really hungry or just bored?" Have fun with it and write sentences will resonate with you.

Stick to unprocessed foods – Foods which are as close to their natural states as possible are best for you and will give you longer lasting energy and a sense of fullness for longer. Switch to wholegrain options; add lots of salads with each meal (simple dressings though – extra virgin olive oil with lemon juice is my favourite) and lots of colourful and leafy vegetables. It might not be sexy to say this stuff, but by eating it, it will help you stay sexy!

Introduce more raw (or lightly cooked) foods – Cooking foods actually destroys vitamins, anti-oxidants, enzymes and essential fatty acids in the foods, so put as much raw food or lightly cooks foods onto your food roster. Something like a vegetable stir-fry is great. It takes less than five minutes to do and is tasty and easy – perfect for those with busy lives. Give salad a starring role on the plate and not just the supporting act – make most of your plate contain salad and give less space to meat and potatoes. You'll still get the flavour of your meal, and will be doing yourself a favour in the long run.

Put your cutlery down between bites – Or put your sandwich or burger down if you're not using cutlery. It seems like it's too simple an idea to work, but if you do that, not only will you tend to spend more time chewing (and thus releasing the enzymes from your mouth) but you'll also be consciously thinking about your food in a more active way and giving your body a chance to catch up with your brain over how much you need to eat.

Use the kitchen table just for eating – Having a dedicated area just for eating will get you into the right frame of mind for this important activity. If you sit in front of the TV with your food, (1) you're probably not sitting with the best posture to digest food properly and (2) you'll also more than likely overeat as you continue to eat to fit in with the length of time of the TV show. By having a dedicated eating spot, you will condition yourself to sit and eat at that spot. If you start doing other things at the dining table you will find that the two activities merge. For example, if you are doing work at the dining table, unconsciously your mind starts to get feelings of food as it associates the table with eating. Better to have a dedicated work area and a dedicated eating area.

Out of sight, out of mind – I used to have trouble restraining myself from over-eating any treats that I would buy. Generally though, I just don't buy them anymore and that's the best option. If you *do* need to have some treats available then make it an effort for you to get to them. Put them right at the back of the cupboard or in the garage or basement tucked away so you forget that they're even there. You might want to have them for when you have visitors round but it doesn't mean that they need to be in your line of sight day-in, day-out. Make it as much of a challenge as possible to get to them.

Plan your meals – If you plan your meals ahead of time, you're less likely to go a grab whatever is quick and easy in front of you. A little bit of planning ahead will ensure that you are consciously thinking about what you will be eating rather than being a slave to the hunger demons.

Graze don't guzzle – Have a supply of decent grazing foods close by such as nuts and seeds. And keep them in your line of sight when working, so that you can grab them when you need to. If they're tucked away in your drawer, you're more likely to make a dash for the vending machine or corner shop.

Distract yourself – Often hunger is a sign of boredom so do some other activity for 5 to 10 minutes instead of the one you might be doing and then come back to it. You will find that a break from the routine and environment will actually make you forget that you were "hungry".

Go small – Serve your food on smaller plates. I used to eat a massive plate of pasta before I made a simple switch and started putting my pasta in a nice little serving bowl. It means I eat less and I still feel satisfied because I've eaten all (or most of) the meal and it's also the way pasta is meant to be served so as to keep the food hotter for longer. The same goes for noodles.

Good. Well I hope these tips will prove to be useful to you. They really are quick and painless to do and *will* make a difference to you in the long term. I promise.

Right now I have a question for you. What comes to mind when you read and think about the word breakfast; or lunch; or dinner? For each of those words I'm sure you get some kind of image. It might be an image of you dashing out in the morning with a slice of toast in your hand and your bag in the other while simultaneously waving goodbye to your spouse and/or kids. Lunch might bring a picture to your mind of eating a popular sandwich chain's special at your desk while answering emails. For the word dinner you might see yourself feeling tired from battling with your commute home, annoyed at having to cook something from scratch and the time it will take when all you want to do is collapse in front of the TV.

Take some time now and close your eyes and think of one of those mealtimes? Do it now....... What feelings came up for you?

For me, when I think of dinner, I get an image of family life and everyone preparing to get ready to talk about their day. I also get a sense that dinner is an opportunity for me to relax and be creative. This stems from the fact that growing up; evening mealtime in my family was always a family affair with my dad usually taking the reins on cooking the evening meal. For my dad, it's a pleasurable experience to cook in the evening – a chance for him to relax and unwind from the day.

I have also inherited that approach but for me it's also a little more about feeling creative (and doing so with speed); whereas my dad prefers to take a good hour or two to prepare the evening spread. I like to be a lot quicker as I'm limited for time in the evenings. Sometimes I don't even know exactly what it is I'll be cooking until I look in my fridge or cupboard and see what I can 'create' from what's in there. Not something I particularly endorse, as by not planning your meals you will have a tendency not to eat as well and put on weight. It's an approach that works for me nevertheless once you know which of your 'staple' ingredients you have lying around work well together. By staple ingredients, for me it's things like onions, lemons, tinned tomatoes, salt, pepper, olive oil, herbs, spices, rice, noodles, pasta, garlic, ginger – these kind of ingredients. Foods that don't spoil quickly, which you can have lying around for ages. It's easy enough to then add a few vegetables in the mix along with some of these essentials to create something really tasty. Many times I have created dishes that I have absolutely loved, but then never cooked again. Mainly because I made no note of what I was doing and was just 'in flow', as they say.

The point is this though. What comes to *your* mind when you think of preparing food? How about when you think of popping round to a friend's place for dinner? Is the image different? In your (home) image; are you seeing yourself stressed out, rushing around trying to do a million different things at once? And in the image of going to your friends; are you surrounded by pleasant smells and a neat and organised kitchen and relaxing atmosphere?

I'm sure you all have your own versions of the above but my point is that how we think about the situation will also determine how we feel about doing that activity. Is it a chore or a pleasure?

A quick way to get yourselves thinking about this differently is to use the 'Swish Pattern' technique you learnt earlier (and repeated below for ease). Again, you might want to get a friend to help guide you through this. If you'd rather work alone then please head to http://thethoughtgym.com/book for the guided support.

Swish Pattern Technique

1. Think of the image that comes to your mind when you think of that meal.

2. Associate into that image – in other words, if you're not already looking through your own eyes, step into the image and notice how you feel.

3. OK, step out and clear the screen. Open your eyes and think of something else. What was the last movie you saw?

4. Now create a new image that will make you really want to cook and prepare a decent meal or sit down and eat your lunch in a relaxing manner.

5. Be fully associated (look through your own eyes) into the image – notice the colours, sounds, feelings that you have.

6. Good, now step out of the image – still holding the image in your mind but so that you can now see yourself in the image.

7. OK, break your state and think of something else. What was the last song you bought?

8. Bring back the image from steps 1 and 2. Now fully associate back into it.

9. Insert a small dark picture of the desired state from step 6 into the lower left corner of the other image.

10. Make sure you can see yourself in that little image.

11. Now for the swish part.

12. While making a swish sound, simultaneously have your desired state (the one from step 6) get bigger and brighter while at the same time have your present image (from step 1) become small and shrink into nothing in the lower left hand corner.

13. Open your eyes and clear your mind. Think of something else. Who's your favourite music artist?

14. Repeat steps 8 to 13 again, this time a little faster.

15. Keep on repeating steps 8-14, getting faster and faster each time. Do this for maybe 5 minutes or at least 15 times, remembering to break your state after each time and clear your mind.

16. Once you've done it at least 15 times, now try and think of that mealtime and see what image comes to mind. Does the old image even appear, or is the change so fast that the new desired image appears?

17. If not, go back and repeat the process until you get it. It takes a bit of practice at first because it's something new and different, so as before, persevere with it.

Wow! Now there was a chapter and a half! I hope you got through it OK and remember that my intention is for you to take your time and learn as much as you can by actively participating in the processes I give you. Well done for getting to this point as you're over half way now and there's still more fun to be had and exciting things to learn.

Chapter Summary

- ✓ Overeating and binge eating are emotionally driven events.
- ✓ You learnt 'anchoring' and Swish pattern techniques that you can use to overcome some unhelpful emotional tendencies.
- ✓ Vegetables are a rich source of protein.
- ✓ Reducing or eliminating meat and dairy from your diets can produce numerous benefits.
- ✓ Many famous and great leaders of the past have been vegetarians.
- ✓ You picked up several tips on how to make small changes to your routine which will yield huge gains.

---

8 - Water

"Water is the driving force of all nature." - Leonardo da Vinci

"We forget that the water cycle and the life cycle are one." – *Jacques Cousteau*

One easy (and essential) action that everyone can do is to drink more water. Water is the key to life on Earth - but it's easy to forget that. The sad fact of the matter is that most people walk around all day in a permanent state of dehydration. If you start to feel thirsty then it's already too late – you're already dehydrated and even slight dehydration can cause your metabolism to slow down. Not good if you're looking to achieve your target weight range, right?

Our bodies are approximately 75% water and so it stands to reason that 75% of our diet should contain water-based foods. Think about everything that you've eaten in the last 24 hours. How much of it was rich in water? Foods like fruits, vegetables, herbal teas and water itself, of course. Meats have next to no water in them and I don't count black teas and coffees as they are actually diuretics and do not add to overall water content.

Our brains are in fact 85% water and so what is often mistaken for hunger is actually dehydration. Keeping yourself hydrated should be your first port of call when it comes to staving off the hunger pangs. If you feel hungry, reach for water first. Even if it isn't dehydration, the water will fill your belly for long enough in order to get something decent, instead of reaching for the first thing that's there. I must point out here though, that although you should consume a good amount of water each day, the best thing would be to balance that out with water-rich foods, like fruits, vegetables and sprouts. It would be no good overloading yourself with water as this can do as much damage as having too little. As a guide, I tend to have between 2 and 4 litres a day. Usually it's around the 3 litre mark although if I'm doing a fair bit of exercise it will be considerably more. How can you get through that much water a day though - especially if you're not into it in the first place? Here are some tips to increase your water intake:

Keep a bottle of water by your bed – First thing in the morning you are dehydrated as you sweat out a lot overnight. Just put your mattress on the floor one night and feel the underneath of it the next morning when the water loss hasn't had a chance to evaporate and you'll understand what I mean. Gulp down a large glass of water to kick start your day.

Have a bottle of water on your desk or close by at all times – If you work at a desk then by having a bottle constantly in front of you it will remind you to drink. And by not having to get up each time to fill a small cup when you want a drink, you'll take more in. I recommend using a 1 litre bottle. This way you can measure how much you drink and make it a goal to drink one bottle in the morning and one in the afternoon. If you do that then coupled with drinking water when you wake up and also when you get home, you should easily meet 3 litres a day. If you think 1 litre in the morning/afternoon sounds too much, just remember to take sips every now and then – perhaps when on the phone and the other person is speaking, or when opening and reading your emails.

Flavour your water – If you find that you don't really like the taste of water, try adding some flavour to it by putting lemon juice in it. I have a lemon corer which inserts right into the lemon and squeezes out the juice without any mess. I recommend getting a metal one as the plastic ones break when you start to squeeze the lemon too hard. There are also plenty of bottled water options with flavourings. I personally prefer to flavour my water with natural lemon instead of bottled lemon juice or to drinking flavoured water, as these sometimes contain other unnecessary ingredients such as potassium metabisulphite (E224) in the case of bottled lemon juice.

Buy a water bottle – Buy a re-usable and BPA-free water bottle. BPA (Bisphenol A) is found in many plastics although the use of it is banned in baby bottles as it is thought to be toxic. If you re-use water bottles which are meant for single use, then they may contain toxins that you wouldn't want in your body. Better to buy a BPA-free bottle. Even better, if you can get one with a built-in filter (I personally use one called a Bobble) then go for that, as the quality of most water leaves a lot to be desired.

Some people when I encourage them to drink lots of water complain that they'll have to keep getting up from their desks to go to the toilet. "Well," I say, "that's a good thing, isn't it? You get to stretch your legs every so often and move your eyes away from the screen." The one thing that I'm big on, and I'll mention it again in a later chapter, is taking small incremental steps. Your goal of achieving your target weight range is like training for a marathon and not a sprint – and furthermore the *maintenance* of your target weight range should be seen as a lifelong journey, so I'm all in favour of small steps to get there. Just do them every day and you will notice changes.

The problem today is that everyone is looking for the quick-fix solution to their problems and not willing to invest the time or energy needed to reach their goals. Just by getting up and going to the toilet every hour or so will mean you probably take an extra 500 - 1000 steps a day, so in my opinion it's worth it for that alone.   Trust me when I say that it's all the small actions combined together that will be the 'difference that makes the difference'. In fact, research is now catching up with me and showing that if you perform N.E.A.T exercises (which stands for Non-Exercise Activity Thermogenesis), you burn a lot more calories each day. N.E.A.T is any activity that you wouldn't normally consider exercise – including getting up from your desk regularly to pop to the toilet!

Not only will consuming water ensure that you keep hydrated and keep the hunger pangs at bay, but consuming water will also mean that you'll be cutting down on all the other liquids that you might drink like your sugar based sodas or coffees.

Another reason why drinking more water is good for you is that it will actually speed up your metabolic rate as your body works to process the water. Researchers at the University of Utah discovered that volunteers who drank eight to twelve glasses of water a day had higher metabolic rates than those who drank only four glasses.

If you're thirsty, then water at room temperature is better to quench your thirst, as the body doesn't need to do much to it before it gets absorbed. Cold water on the other hand needs to be warmed up by the body first, before you reap the full benefits, but it actually helps you burn more calories. Not many, but they all add up. The reason for this is as follows. If you take a 250 ml glass of ice water it weighs 250g. Because it takes 1 calorie to raise 1 gram of water by 1 degree Celsius, to make that water reach your body temperature of 37 degrees Celsius, it would need to expend just over 9 Calories. This is calculated from 250g x 37 degrees = 9250 calories. Remembering that a food Calorie (Calorie – with a capital C) is actually equivalent to a kilocalorie, gives us a figure of 9 Calories. It doesn't sound like much, but if you have 10 glasses a day, then that's an extra 90 Calories (*each day*) for not doing anything extra. That's over 30,000 extra calories a year used, or almost 4kg! Personally I don't recommend drinking ice cold water all the time, but even if it's not that cold, you get the picture.

Some people complain that they have water retention and restrict the amount of water they drink. The thing is, your body is smart and realises when it's being starved of water and so will retain what it can – in the same way that it has the capability to get rid of any excess. The less water you drink, the more the body will retain, so you're better off getting your body used to the idea that it has a plentiful supply of water and it will soon learn to flush away the reserves that it stores. It might also be worth checking your salt intake if you're storing lots of water, as the body tends to hold on to water in order to dilute the excess salt.

Water really is the elixir of life. Your skin will look better, younger and you will feel more energised while having greater levels of concentration. There is so much that can be written about this magical substance that it deserves a whole book in itself and I simply don't have the space here. If there's one thing that you take away from this book it would be to make sure you get enough good quality water each and every day.

Chapter Summary

✓ Our bodies are around 75% water and our brains are about 85%.
✓ Most people are in a constant state of dehydration.
✓ Dehydration is often misinterpreted by the brain as hunger, so drink first.
✓ Drink between 2-4 litres of water a day.
✓ Keep a bottle of water close by for frequent top ups throughout the day.
✓ Staying well hydrated will speed up your metabolism, make your skin look healthier and younger and will keep you from overeating.

9 - Exercise

"No man has the right to be an amateur in the matter of physical training. It is a shame for a man to grow old without seeing the beauty and strength of which his body is capable." - Socrates

"Lack of activity destroys the good condition of every human being, while movement and methodical physical exercise save it and preserve it." - Plato

When it comes to being on top of your health and weight issues, there's one thing that you can't avoid – exercise. Statistics show that somehow 39% of adults manage to avoid even setting foot in a gym since leaving school! And a common excuse for not exercising is "I don't have time". Well, you know what the great leveller for all of us is? The thing that makes us all equal – no matter race, religion, finances or status? It's that we all have 24hrs in a day. If successful (and really busy) people like a Richard Branson or a Barack Obama can 'find' time to stay healthy while running multi-billion pound companies and global superpowers, do you think that you might also be able to 'find' the time too? I say 'find' in quotes, as you can't really 'find' any more time. There are still only 24hrs in a day – no matter how hard you look! In reality, you're going to have to 'take' time. Take it from somewhere else: watching TV, surfing online, lying in bed or some other activity. Be honest with yourself and know that if your life depended on it (and it might well do), you would 'take' the time from somewhere.

Why *should* you exercise though? Well aside from burning the fuel that you consume, exercise will strengthen your bones, your heart and your lungs. By being fit and healthy you will be able to pump more oxygen around your body and give your cells more oxygen and thus more energy. Exercise also releases endorphins (the body's natural 'feel good' chemicals) which make you feel great. Exercise will also boost your immune system helping you fight off illness and make you less susceptible to getting ill in the first place. Another great reason to exercise is to release tension and stress which gets built up as part of your body's natural defence mechanism. When you encounter some kind of threat (and it can be either physical or emotional – your body doesn't distinguish between the two) your body prepares to deal with it. It does this by releasing your 'fight or flight' response thinking it needs to run away or take some kind of action. If this 'fight or flight' response is activated but then has no means by which to dissipate, then it will get stored up as tension. By engaging in regular exercise this build up of tension and stress has an outlet.

Ideally your exercise routine should combine aerobic exercise – that's the kind which makes you huff and puff a bit - with strength training. Strength or resistance training being activities like push ups, squats, weight training, BodyPump™ and so on. Strength training is important as it actually helps burn fat faster by boosting your metabolism. For every 450g of muscle you have, you burn through an additional 50 calories a day – for doing essentially nothing! Not only that, strength training also increases bone density helping prevent osteoporosis, lowers your blood pressure and cholesterol levels. By preventing these conditions strength training will help to lower the risk of stroke, diabetes, cancer and arthritis. Add to that an increase in energy levels, better moods (remember the extra endorphins) and sleep patterns, and there really is no reason *not* to do it.

And it gets better. The good news is that exercise is all around you and the majority of you out there are doing it all the time anyway. You just haven't been calling it that. Whenever you are doing some form of activity that gets you to breathe heavier and more rapidly than you are at rest; *that* is a form of exercise. The trick here is how to incorporate more of it into your day. And it gets even better. By simply realising that the tasks you do on a daily basis can be considered a form of exercise, and knowing how many calories you burn doing them will actually help you in your weight maintenance.

This was shown to be the case in a Harvard University study by Alia Crum and Ellen Langer as reported in Richard Wiseman's book, 59 Seconds. Crum and Langer asked themselves what would happen to people if you told them that their job was actually considered exercise. Would it make a difference to their weight and blood pressure?

They used two groups of hotel attendants as the sample groups. One group were told nothing and the other were told how many calories they used doing each of their daily tasks. After Crum and Langer returned a month later, they found that the control group had no change in weight or blood pressure but the other group had lost a significant amount of weight and lowered their blood pressure. And that's without doing anything extra. Just realising that they were in fact exercising was enough to help them lose weight. Crum and Langer believed it was to do with the placebo effect and that by knowing they were exercising the attendants changed their beliefs about themselves. Of course, you now already know just how powerful beliefs and belief changes can be, after having worked through this book up to here.

I go to the gym quite frequently, but I didn't always; and I was still happy about how I felt and looked. This was because I did other things that would help me stay fit and remain active. I'm not a real believer either in having to be super sporty or a gym bunny in order to be fit and healthy. I incorporate exercise where I can. If I encounter a flight of stairs I take them (and two at a time to really work into the thighs, butt and abs). If it's a choice between a short bus or tube journey and a walk - I choose the walk. Examine your day-to-day routines and identify or create opportunities around you to exercise without paying for a gym membership or joining a club or slogging it out running round the park. I mentioned N.E.A.T. in the previous chapter which is basically showing that anything active will count. Just walking at a modest 1.5 miles per hour will increase your metabolism by 100% compared to sitting – so next time you're on your mobile phone to your friends, get 'mobile' yourself!

One of the best forms of exercise is walking. If you can fit in ten to twelve thousand steps a day, the chances are that you're not overweight. Many studies have attempted to quantify what the magic number is for the number of steps an average person should take a day. A frequently cited number is 10,000 steps but I would suggest that you should really be aiming for even more than that – nearer to 12,000.

A study performed by Dr James Hill, director of the Colorado Nutrition Obesity Research Centre, noted that the average number of steps taken each day by women between the ages of 18 – 50 was 5000 steps and for men 6000 steps. Interestingly though, the study revealed that people who were considered overweight, took 1500-2000 fewer steps than their healthy weight counterparts. Imagine that. The difference between being overweight or not is only 2000 steps a day – or about a mile. Isn't that fascinating? So if you aim to complete 10,000 – 12,000 steps a day, I suspect that you will be fine. Of course we're all different and what's true for one person might not be true for another, so buy a pedometer and gauge where you are now (both during the week and also at weekends, as the number will vary). Commit to increasing your daily step count by 500 steps a week until you reach 10 – 12,000. If you're still overweight at that point, consider increasing that number but more importantly really examine what you're fuelling those 12,000 steps with.

Here are some tips to incorporate more walking into your life:

➤ Take a walk with your friends or family to talk about the day instead of doing it while the TV is on.

➤ Take a 3 minute walking 'air' break instead of a cigarette break – you'll be outside anyway.

➤ Walk every chance you get – for example at the shops, park in the furthest space from the store and not the closest. You'll get out of the car park quicker when they're busy too.

➤ Walk off any stressful situations and allow your 'fight or flight' instinct to take flight. It will also clear your head and enable you to come at the problem from a different and potentially more creative angle.

➤ Take the stairs between floors at your place of work. Even if it's only a floor or two, it will all add up. And if it's more than that then you don't have to take the lift for all of them. Take it half way in the beginning and work up to it.

Just take an inventory of where you are now and decide to make small incremental improvements. You don't have to do everything all at once. I find with many clients that they can become overwhelmed with the task required, and focus too much on wanting to do everything, believing it's just too much. Other people initially like the challenge and go for it full throttle only to lose enthusiasm for it later on. If you build up gradually you're more likely to condition both your mind and body into the kind of changes I'm describing in this book. After all, *how do you eat an elephant?* Well, one bite at a time of course!

I love walking around London as it's often the best mode of transport available. It also lets me take time to really look at and appreciate the architecture. That's walking, but do you know what the best exercise is for getting fit and reaching your target weight?

Whichever one you're going to stick to! There are a number of different activities that qualify as exercise and it's not just the regular ones like running, swimming, cycling and football. How about dog-walking, Frisbee, rollerblading, gardening, painting, Salsa, Zumba... Here's a list of exercises that I personally enjoy doing, together with my thoughts on them.

> **Running** – Great for noticeable improvements in short periods of time. The downside is that each heel strike puts about 4x your body weight through the knees and ankles and over time injuries can hit you. Stretching is essential to prevent your muscles from getting too tight because if you neglect stretching, I promise you, you *will* suffer. That said; a great run can release an endorphin high that will keep you wanting to do more. Make sure you go to a dedicated running shop (and not a normal high street shop catering for the fashion connoisseur's trainers) and get your trainers properly fitted. Some will film you running and examine your running style and

recommend appropriate trainers for you in order to prevent injuries and make running more enjoyable. Perhaps investigate the latest approach (cited to prevent injuries) – barefoot running.

Swimming – A great example for overall muscle tone and fitness if done properly. The buoyancy of the water supports your body and reduces the risk of injury. Although getting to a decent pool can be a challenge, and results may be less speedy than with running, it's a worthwhile exercise. I often use swimming as a way of staying in shape when I'm injured. And if you're not a fan of swimming, how about giving Aqua-aerobics a go? I used to do my own version of this whenever I was on holiday in Cyprus (long before Aqua-aerobics was on any gym timetables). I would be in the sea and perform all manner of exercises under the surface of the water. Treading water by mimicking running, weird Tai chi-style arm and leg motions, all whilst having the sea provide resistance for me. I would do anything fun I could think of and best of all, from the shore it just looked like I was treading water like anyone else!

Cycling – I still cycle but primarily only as a mode of transport. There's less impact on the joints, it gets you around in a quick and guaranteed fashion and is both environmentally and financially friendly. On the flip side, you need to make time for stretching - it's essential to make time for stretching after exercising; otherwise not only do you risk injury but you'll also tighten your muscles and restrict your range of movement. In addition, the lactic acid built up in the muscles during exercise won't be able to dissipate properly if you don't stretch. If you decide to cycle to work for instance, consider where and how you will store your gear and whether there is somewhere to change and shower. Having access to showers and changing rooms just depends on your individual commute and might not be necessary for you, so perhaps just give cycling a go and see if it works for your routine. Just *decide* to do it and then any barriers you thought were there will soon tumble as you find answers to overcome them.

Rebounding – This is one of my favourite exercises as it's quick and easy to do. A rebounder is essentially a mini-trampoline that you bounce up and down on. A variety of rebounders are on the market, but I recommend spending what you can in order to get the best quality and durability. I use a Bellicon® rebounder and can certainly recommend it. The jumping surface is connected with bungee cords (instead of springs) so is not only silent but also softer on the joints than spring counterparts. That said, there are other ones which have springs which are good too – just be considerate if you have neighbours downstairs if you live in a flat! Rebounding is great. You can do it in the comfort of your own home, while watching TV, talking on the phone or just thinking. I find that rebounding wakes me up perfectly in the mornings and stimulates all the right cells in my body ready for the day and it engages all 638 muscles in your body. It doesn't require much time each day either. I would start with 5 minutes and, depending on how much time you have, increase this incrementally to 15 - 30 minutes. You'll be amazed at the results after just a short period of time.

Yoga - The one exercise that I totally recommend for everyone is yoga. I've been doing it on and off now for over 8 years and more regularly for the last 5 years. I have to say that it's the one exercise I would always want to keep doing because of all the benefits; from becoming stronger and more flexible, to learning about the power of the breath and aiding relaxation. I would warn you though, it can take time to really 'get into it' - but it's worth it. Like I said, I've been doing it quite a while now and I'm still learning things all the time.

Here's why I'm so into yoga. In 2008, I went to see a neck specialist because of an ongoing neck problem. I was constantly in pain and I found it extremely difficult to rotate my neck to the side. The MRI showed I had a compressed disc in my neck and I was told about three ways in which I could have it treated, which were: to operate, get an injection or do physiotherapy. I opted for physiotherapy as injections seemed to me to be just a fancy pain killer, treating the symptom rather than the cause and an operation seemed too invasive. I wanted to solve the root cause of the issue and felt non-intrusive action was the way to go. The physiotherapy worked well, but as with anything, if you don't use it you lose it. So in order to maintain good posture and movement I got more serious about yoga. I'm pleased to say that my neck is a lot better these days and I absolutely know that yoga played a massive part. Not only in performing the exercises themselves, but also allowing me to become more aware of my body. I notice that if I don't go for a while, the pain and movement becomes worse.

Another key reason for me practicing yoga is to support the continuous rehabilitation of my shoulder injury (the snowboarding one I mentioned earlier). Doctors advised me that I'm now more likely to develop arthritis in that shoulder because of the injury, but I know that with constant exercise supplemented by a good diet, I'm at least stacking the cards in my favour. Let me also tell you something else that gets me into that class. When I think of growing older, not having maintained regular yoga practice, I have images pop into my mind of not being able to put my socks on without supporting myself against something. Weird, I know. But I do think about that sort of stuff! Also, whenever I see a more 'mature' person with curvature in their back, neck and shoulders, it serves to remind me why I'm doing all this – to give myself the best possible chance of being mobile and active in the future.

In practicing yoga, you probably won't shed the pounds as quickly as with some other forms of exercise but you will notice the difference after only a few visits. You must be patient with yoga and also resist the temptation to compare yourself to others. Yoga is quite a personal journey into your own mind-body connection and everyone progresses at a pace that suits them. Hunt around for good instructors and I encourage you to seek out proper yoga studios as opposed to gym yoga classes as gyms tend to (in my experience) have shorter and less in depth classes. That said; I was fortunate to find a gym yoga class that was a decent length (1.5 hours) and with a very knowledgeable and great instructor – thanks Charlie!

I also do a number of other activities ranging from BodyPump™, circuit training and Pilates to hiking, canoeing and mountain biking. The thing is this - find something that you like doing and do that. It's not all about gyms, clubs or team sports. Just add more and more activity into your day consistently and you will notice measureable results. There are always opportunities around us to move our bodies more. It can be simple; walking the dog, mowing the lawn, cleaning the house or simply deciding to walk up escalators instead of standing on the right with everyone else. Sticking with the majority also gives you what the majority have. That is: poor exercise regimes, being overweight and languishing from a lack of energy.

So how much should you exercise? I would recommend that you do what you can, from where you are now, and work up to 4 -6 times a week; a mixture of 30-40 minute sessions of aerobic exercise and resistance training. By aerobic I mean that you're at a training intensity whereby it's possible to sustain a conversation but it's not easy. You don't want to be so out of breath that you enter the anaerobic training zone, but not have it so easy that you're barely raising your heart rate.

You must spend time warming up in order to gradually raise your heart rate and wake up your muscles to prevent injury (about 12 minutes) and also warm down (about 5-10 minutes) and then stretch. I've mentioned it before but it's worth re-stating because I see so many people training who think that stretching is a luxury if time allows. No. It's vitally important that you plan for stretching to be part of your workout as not only will it prevent injury, increase your range of movement and dissipate lactic acid build up, but it will also lengthen your muscles allowing more of the muscle to benefit from the workout (and up to 30% of the benefits of your workout could be lost if you don't stretch).

I perform dynamic stretching at the beginning of a workout (after the warm up) and static stretching at the end of the workout (after the warm down). Dynamic stretching is where you exaggerate the movements you are likely to perform in the main exercise rather than holding just a position. Static stretching is where an adopted position is held for a particular length of time. I recommend holding the stretch for as many seconds as you are old and then swapping sides and repeating. So, being 35, I would hold a quad stretch, as an example, for 35 seconds and then swap sides before performing a second round of quad stretching. This book is designed to give you a feel for how to get into exercise and the mindset you need. To ensure maximum benefit of any exercise program, I recommend that you seek professional advice when starting out.

A good investment would be to purchase a simple heart rate monitor for use while exercising. One with a stopwatch, current heart rate, average heart rate and perhaps some audible sound alerts when in and out of target heart rate range should suffice. Without a heart rate monitor you can always use the Rate of Perceived Exertion (RPE) heart rate method. This is to listen to your body really and *perceive* how hard you are working using the ten point scale below.

> ➤ RPE 1-2:Very easy; you can converse with no effort

> ➤ RPE 3: Easy; you can converse with almost no effort

> ➤ RPE 4: Moderately easy; you can converse comfortably with little effort

> ➤ RPE 5: Moderate; conversation requires some effort

> ➤ RPE 6: Moderately hard; conversation requires quite a bit of effort

> ➤ RPE 7: Difficult; conversation requires a lot of effort

> ➤ RPE 8: Very difficult; conversation requires maximum effort

> ➤ RPE 9-10:   Peak effort; no-talking zone

A good level would be around 6 or 7 if you're used to exercising, otherwise aim for level 5. From level 7 onwards, you're really moving towards *an*aerobic (without oxygen) training and there's no real need to head there for the purposes of this book.

If you do have (or purchase) a heart rate monitor then you can use the simple formula of 220 minus your age to get your maximum heart rate and work out a percentage from there (60%-70% ideally).

For a 35 year old, that would be between 111 and almost 130 beats per minute (bpm).

220 – 35 = 185 MAXIMUM HEART RATE

60 % of 185 = 111

70% of 185 = 129.5

Here are some top exercise tips I use which may be useful to you. The good news is that research shows that if you get into the habit of exercising *consistently* for 6 months, then you are more likely to stick with it and even return to it after any significant absences. Less than this period of time, and the habit of exercising is easy to forget.

1. **Pre-pack your kit** – Pre-pack your kit bag the day (or several days) before. I often pack my bag for the Monday on the preceding Friday when I get home so that I know it's done and if anything distracts me on the weekend I'm still good to go on Monday morning. This way your bag is ready for when you need it and you won't have those last minute excuses. Also, have a dedicated kit bag which will have all your necessary toiletries, padlocks, water bottles and anything else. Buy doubles of all your toiletries so you don't need to keep moving things around from bathroom to bag and back again.

2. **Timetable your workouts** - Book the time for your workouts in your calendar. I have a weekly planner on my fridge which has all my weekly commitments already populated. I also have my workouts as recurring meetings in my Microsoft 'Outlook' calendar. This means that whenever I get something from the fridge or open my Outlook calendar I consciously (and unconsciously) see the training schedule in there and I get reminded to go. I can also keep track of when I went to the gym (as I delete out the entries if I miss a session). This can serve as a great reminder to show you how much you've done. Not only this, but if it's blocked out in your calendar then other people won't be able to schedule time in with you and interrupt your routine. Furthermore, once it's written down it becomes a commitment that you've made to yourself. When we really commit to ourselves we actually feel quite uncomfortable breaking it. Have you ever been invited to a party that you weren't really keen on going to and so have answered that you will "try and make it", or "hope to make it", or will "aim to be there". It's better because it lets you off the hook if you don't go. As soon as you commit and say you *will* be there, suddenly everything changes. You feel compelled to make it there and make it happen.

3. **Incorporation** - We all lead busy lives and so take an inventory of your daily routine and determine where you can increase your exercise activity. It might be simply to walk up the stairs instead of taking the lift, get off the bus or underground a stop earlier, or walk home with the shopping bags instead of going for the taxi. As an illustration of how even walking home with the shopping can turn into a mini workout; my walk from the local

mini-market is about 5 minutes and so by carrying a couple of bags in each arm I'm able to do some bicep curls en route home!

4. **Plan your workouts/exercise** - Make the best use of your time and efforts and plan what you're going to do before you do it and you can cut the total amount of exercise time down. A lot of time is wasted when people head off to the gym with no real plan about what they are going to do or they idly stand by waiting to use a machine - so have a backup plan as well. I go to classes regularly and there have been many times when something prevents me from attending. It might be cancelled, already full or I'm delayed and miss too much to join in. For the times when I don't fancy a main gym floor workout, I make sure that I have my swimming kit permanently in my bag and I go for a dip instead. Especially if it's before work, as it's a great way to wake up and feel energised. I often follow a swim with 10 minutes in the steam room – wonderful!

5. **Train with music** – A study from Dr Michael Miller of the University of Maryland determined that listening to upbeat music improved the ability of blood vessels to expand 30% as blood passed through them which may be why other studies have shown that you exercise an additional 30% longer if you have some tunes to motivate you along the way. Depending on the training, you'll want to adapt the music. Perhaps a nice steady beat for running or something really motivational for the end of a hard workout. I personally think you can't go wrong with the Rocky soundtrack. It gets me every time!

6. **Train with friends** - If you can train with a buddy then you'll enjoy it more and also feel a sense of commitment to the process so will be more inclined to stick with it. It's much harder to let someone else down than yourself plus you'll get to spend more time with your friends and strengthen your relationship.

7. **Make use of the sauna and steam rooms** - If you're training in a gym, then make use of these little gems. It will relax you of course - but more importantly it will help elevate your heart rate and in turn your metabolism; sweat out toxins and, provided it's quiet and there's enough space, give you the perfect place to perform deep stretching. Remember to take a large bottle of water in there and make sure you drink just as much water as you lose.

8. **Use your imagination** - When I'm doing an activity, I find that it helps if I visualise something while doing it. So if I'm in the pool swimming; in my head I'm swimming in the Mediterranean. If I'm on the treadmill, then I'm running on the streets completing a race to roaring crowds. When I'm on my bike around London, often I imagine being on a race round the city competing against others on the hunt for some prize. It can be anything which will make your activity more enjoyable.

At this point, I would like to mention something about some of the concepts in this book. They do involve a change of routine slightly and what you're used to. I understand that. And in my experience, people often resist change - at least when it's not *their* idea. And even sometimes when they know that change is good for them, people still resist. The thing is that we often try to change too much too soon. I recommend making small changes initially, even if they seem inconsequential at first. You might argue that you can't see the point of the suggestions you're about to read below, but let me tell you why they *are* important. Firstly, they will get you used to change and the idea that change isn't necessarily a bad thing. Secondly, by making a change to a habitual pattern, you become more aware of your actions and are able to realise whether any improvements can be made. And lastly, ultimately, these techniques re-wire the connections in your brain and increase your capacity for change.

Here are some suggestions on how to make small changes to your daily routine. These may feel strange initially, but they will train you to the notion that change is OK.

1. **Change your walk to work** - Do you always walk the same way to work? Cross at the same crossing? I found that when I changed this each day or every few days I became less like a robot and more conscious about my journey. It felt odd, but somehow refreshing to catch myself thinking "No, I'm going to take the left hand route today".

2. **Putting trousers on** - Do you always put a certain leg through first? I tend to favour one leg over the other. I think it's important to become aware of this and change things from time to time. It also makes you look at other areas of life where you are perhaps doing things just out of habit and without much thought. Give it a go and see what it feels like to mix things up every now and then.

3. **Shaving** - I used to always have a set pattern for how I shaved. Starting with the upper lip area and then going to the right cheek, then neck, then left and then finally the chin. I realised I was doing it the same way *every* time. When I changed the order around, it felt weird at first. The aim here is to get comfortable with the uncomfortable.

4. **Brushing your teeth** - Like the shaving, do you always brush in a certain way? Mix it up a little, and also brush with the opposite hand now and then too. How does that feel?

The objective of all this is to get you *used* to being comfortable with change and comfortable with the uncomfortable. Once you do it for small things, your brain will learn that change is okay and that you can still get the results you want and that these results may even be better. We don't have to be fixed into a particular way of behaving and we can actively change how we interpret things – like change. The way the brain and nervous system have evolved means that they are able to change both structurally and functionally as a result of input from the environment – a phenomenon known as neuroplasticity. It is this phenomenon that allows us to re-wire our own brains by what we do and how we think. The study of the birth of neurons (Neurogenesis) is starting to gather evidence that the process of new neurons being created in the brain continues into adulthood. Neurogenesis is important for learning, memory and other cognitive behaviour and the possibility that this process doesn't cease once you become an adult is exciting for me as it means that we're not restricted to how our brains have evolved to date. And what's also interesting, is that Neurogenesis is believed to improve with exercise - yet another reason to exercise. It's a stimulating area of study – and complicated - but effectively, to me it means that you "*can* teach an old dog new tricks".

And what if by changing your walk to work slightly you discover a cool new shop, or bump into an old friend? I have found that, in my experience, many people are just living out their lives day to day, in the same old routine, in a robotic fashion. By living this way, it makes it that much more challenging to introduce new concepts and ideas into the mind. Your mind becomes more like a block of concrete resistant to absorbing new information or changing appearance, than if it were more like a sponge – able to absorb more and change appearance. In order for you to fully appreciate and take advantage of the material in this book, your old way of thinking and habits will have to transform and evolve. Rather than start with the big stuff, start with small things, like a walk to work or brushing your teeth and you will be more open to adapt when it comes to the bigger stuff.

When *should* you exercise?

Well, in short - whatever time works best for you. However, I would recommend, if at all possible, do it first thing in the morning. There are several reasons for this.

1. Your metabolism slows down overnight and so exercising first thing in the morning will give it a kick-start which will keep your metabolic rate optimum and elevated throughout the day.

2. You won't give yourself time to come up with excuses and there's less chance that 'life' will get in the way.

3. Most people will cope fine with a few minutes less sleep so if you can schedule in just 15 minutes in

the morning it won't interrupt your routine too much.

4. You will feel invigorated and energised for the rest of the day and be sharper and more productive as a result, especially if you eat well too.

5. If you commute (especially in London) and can fit it in before work, then by travelling on the tube earlier you'll miss the daily squeeze with the rest of the cattle.

6. According to the University of Delaware's dedicated fitness website, a recent study showed that if you exercise in the morning there's a 75% chance of keeping it up compared to 25% for evening exercisers.

You might be thinking to yourself - "but I'm not a morning person Hari". Well, to tell the truth, neither was I. I had a belief that I simply couldn't exercise in the morning; that I couldn't wake up early enough to do this. I used some of the techniques in this book to change that belief and I'll explain a few of them below.

1. Questions

Instead of making statements like "I can't get up and exercise" or "I'm not a morning person", I asked myself:

➤ *"How can I exercise in the morning and enjoy it?"*

➤ *"What will I need to focus on to get me up in the morning?"*

➤ *"What will it cost me if I don't get up early to exercise?"*

➤ *"What can I do today to move me towards my health and fitness goals?"*

In answering the first question, the answer to me was to attend classes at the gym. I was never into classes before, but the commitment of signing up to them would ensure that I got up. Furthermore, the motivation provided by others and the instructor would get me through it. Knowing that I wasn't alone in this crazy act of morning workouts helped a great deal too!

The answer to my second question was (and still is) that I focus on the end result. When I wake up, I'm thinking of (and visualising, if you will) being in the nice hot shower at the gym *after* the workout and feeling really invigorated and refreshed. I'm not focussing on getting up, or travelling there or anything else; just the feeling of satisfaction at the end of the workout.

My answer to the third question was that if I didn't get up, I would have to travel at rush-hour (no doubt with someone's armpit thrust in my face), I wouldn't be sharp the rest of the day, I would start putting on weight, I would waste my evening if I went after work or worse still; waste my money if I didn't go at all.

Design yourself a series of questions that will help you get up in the morning. As a guide, use the ones above and perhaps some of the ones below. Write down your answers so that they are firmly in your mind and then they will be automatic soon enough.

The Thought Gym

a) *How can I exercise in the morning and enjoy it?*

_____
_____
_____
_____
_____
_____
_____

b) *What will I need to focus on to get me up in the morning?*

_____
_____
_____
_____
_____
_____
_____
_____
_____

c) *What will it cost me if I don't get up early to exercise?*

_____
_____
_____
_____
_____
_____
_____

d) *What am I currently spending time doing in the morning which either can be done later or eliminated altogether?*

_____
_____
_____
_____
_____
_____
_____
_____

e) *What are all the benefits I will get by exercising first thing in the morning?*

_____
_____
_____
_____
_____
_____
_____
_____

2. Better sleep

By incorporating a few things to help me enjoy a better night's sleep I was able to get up with more energy and vitality and therefore have the resources to go to the gym first thing in the morning. There are several rituals that I incorporated which mean I am able to sleep better and fall asleep almost immediately once I climb into bed.

When I was a kid it used to take me anything from 40 minutes to an hour to fall asleep after getting into bed. I would feel quite awake and have thoughts running through my head. I realise now that part of the reason was a habit that my mum had, which was to make us all a cup of tea late at night. Ludicrous when I think about it now, as a cup of tea is precisely what most people drink in the morning to wake them up! A few years ago when I was living in Greece, I was in a dorm room and I didn't have the facilities for tea making (in fact, it's not so common to drink tea out there and so I couldn't easily get my daily cuppa). What I discovered was that when I got back to the UK after getting used to not drinking a cuppa before bed, I was able to sleep a lot better.

Tea drinking is a very British cultural ritual and it's one of these habits that's hard to break for many people. Nowadays, I don't drink any tea or coffee unless it's herbal and the benefits for me personally have been great. I don't need it to wake me up in the morning and if you think about it, if you need some kind of stimulant to keep you awake, something's got to be wrong. You need to look at the causes rather than just addressing the symptoms. It's like trying to mop up the floor when the tap is still left on and the sink is overflowing. Stopping tea and coffee made me feel like a cloud had been lifted from my head and I have become more focussed and sharp as a result. I wasn't even a heavy tea or coffee drinker, so just imagine the difference you would experience if you are a heavy tea or coffee drinker right now. How would you feel if you stopped drinking altogether or reduced your intake? You would probably see even more impressive results than I did. Only you will know for sure, if you give it a go for just a few weeks.

I've digressed a little on the point about sleeping but all these aspects are interlinked. For those of you with children, just think for a second what you do to get your kids off to bed when they're still young? Perhaps you run them a bath, read them a story, get them calmed down before going to bed. And then what do we do as adults? We watch TV, maybe the evening news blasting us with encouraging stories about death, destruction and other joyful events. Maybe we have a drink of alcohol (just to aid the dehydration that is already going to occur overnight) and then we jump straight into bed and wonder why we can't sleep or why we don't sleep enough. Perhaps we should follow the same example that we set for kids?

I've got into the habit of leaving the TV off most evenings. Instead I read, or listen to soft classical music or something else chilled. I sometimes drink a cup of camomile tea and the other thing I did was to turn off the clock in my bedroom so I don't know the exact time when I go to bed – in fact now I've moved it to another room. I do this because often when we go to bed we see the clock and our last thought before closing our eyes might be something like "Oh now, only 'X' hours till I have to get up". This is an unnecessary stress last thing before bed that won't help you sleep. If you decide to follow that example and avoiding the clock time, be mindful of being on the computer last thing at night too, as you'll see the time there too. Another thing that will help you sleep better will be to eat at least 2-3 hours before bed and to have a light meal, so easy on the pasta, rice, meat etc.

Often we might go to bed with many thoughts rushing around our heads about the day, the next day, things we have to do, arguments we've had and so on. If you find yourself in that situation, it will help to write them down. We tend to occupy a lot of our time holding on to things that we really don't need to – just to remember them. By writing them down – be that the list of things to do the following day or any thoughts and conflicts you might have, you release them from your mind and will be able to: 1) focus on them when necessary and with greater clarity because they are written down and 2) you will free up space in your head to relax. I do recommend that approach if you find that that's your problem. Buy a journal or notebook and keep a pen and paper by your bed to jot these down. I've heard it said before that you should never end a day without first planning the next and I think that's true. When we know what we've got to do and have planned it to some degree we feel more comfortable and able to relax.

Another thing that I've found useful to do to really decompress from the day is some mini-meditation. I recommend this as it really does help to unwind. I recommend learning about meditation and how to do some simple techniques but for the purposes here, it's enough just to sit comfortably, with an upright back and close your eyes while focussing on the breath, going in...... and out. It might help for you to say something as it goes in.....and then out again. Or visualise a colour of the breath as it goes in and perhaps a different one as it comes out. Just two or three minutes of that and you will feel the difference. Maybe even work up to 15 – 20 minutes?

3. Visualisation

The next tip for helping you to get up earlier is visualisation. I already mentioned that I visualise myself in the shower *after* already having gone to the gym and completing my workout. Well, before going to bed have a go at doing this. Sit at the end of your bed and with your eyes closed. Imagine that it's the next morning - a minute or two before your alarm is about to wake you up. See yourself lying in bed and really set the scene around you. What can you see and feel? Now associate yourself into the picture and imagine that you're asleep and then imagine as you wake up that you are full of energy and enthusiasm for the day – literally leaping out of bed. The time on the clock by your bed is a minute or two before the time you would normally get up.

Do that just before you go to bed and witness what happens. As you get better about seeing yourself getting up full of energy and enthusiasm, that's just what will happen. And to take it a step further, add what you want to happen from there. For example, imagine yourself waking up and leaping out of bed, heading straight to the bathroom, splashing some water on your face and then heading out to do your exercise (or whatever it might be). Run this through in your mind with vivid clarity and emotion and once you get good at it, it will soon start to become just like your vision. I'm going to talk more about visualisation in a later chapter, so don't worry if you don't get it exactly at this stage.

Some other practical steps you might want to take to get you up and out of bed would be to have a really uplifting and motivating music track as your wake up alarm, or putting your alarm in the adjacent room so you have to get up to turn it off.

I mentioned yoga before and how one of the benefits I found was the breathing aspect of it. Breathing really is the most important thing – getting oxygen to the cells is vital for them to function properly and also to allow the flow of waste to move from your cells via the lymph. Think of the lymph cells like your own private sewage system which is there to remove all the toxins from your cells. The thing with the lymph system is though, that unlike the bloodstream, which has a pump (the heart) the lymph system doesn't and so it needs both movement and deep breathing to stimulate it.

The fact of the matter is that most people don't know how to breathe properly. Sure, you're all out there breathing now but I'm willing to bet that it's shallow, rapid and high up in the chest. A study by lymphologist, Dr Jack Shields from Cottage Hospital in Santa Barbara showed that the most effective way to stimulate the lymph system and get rid of toxins (up to 15 times more efficiently) is to perform deep diaphragmatic breathing exercises regularly. Let me also share with you another bit of information about oxygen and breathing.

Dr Otto Warburg, former director of the Max Plank Institute and two time Nobel Prize winner, conducted experiments with cells and was able to turn healthy cells malignant just by limiting the amount of oxygen that they received.

In his own words Dr Warburg is quoted as saying that *"cancer, above all other diseases, has countless secondary causes. But, even for cancer, there is only one prime cause. Summarized in a few words, the prime cause of cancer is the replacement of the respiration of oxygen in normal body cells by a fermentation of sugar."*

Furthermore, other researchers extended his research and Dr Harry Goldblatt, a recipient of the prestigious Scientific Achievement Award from the American Medical Association, conducted research on cells – some with restricted oxygen and some with normal amounts. After 30 days he injected these cells into groups of rats. The results were shocking. After two weeks – the two normal groups had no change (the ones which were injected with normally oxygenated cells or the control group with no injection). All the rats in third group with the restricted oxygen cells had malignant growths – even after a year the results were the same. I'm not saying this to scare you; more to stress to you just how important getting oxygen via proper breathing is for your health. It's so simple and free!

Whenever I look at the majority of Eastern physical practises such as yoga or martial arts, there is always an emphasis on the power of breathing. There are 75 trillion cells in your body and all of them need food. Their primary food requirement is oxygen and often when you feel tired and lacking in energy, it's not food that you need, but oxygen. Most people breathe from their upper chests and also their breathing tends to be quite short and rapid. What you should be doing is taking fewer and *deeper*, diaphragmatic breaths. Here's an exercise for you to do which will leave you feeling energised and fitter. I learnt this from a training programme by Tony Robbins and have been doing it regularly ever since.

Read the entire process through first and adjust the timings to suit your level of capability, but do push a little bit beyond your comfort zone in order to get the most out of it.

Breathing Process

1. Take a deep breath in - making sure that you fill your stomach first and then raising your chest.

2. Keeping breathing in and count to '4' (seconds).

3. Hold for '16' seconds (4 times the '4' second inhale).

4. Breathe out for '8' seconds (two times the '4' second inhale), really pulling that navel in and towards your spine.

5. Take a normal deep breath.

6. Repeat steps 1 – 5 another 9 times.

7. Do this first thing in the morning, before lunch and before dinner.

If you prefer a guided process of this exercise, go to http://thethoughtgym.com/book.

The ratio of breathing in, holding and then breathing out is 1:4:2 and has been shown to be most effective for stimulating the flow of lymph. You can adjust the time that you breathe in for to a number that you find most comfortable, but stretch yourself. Remember that in order to get stronger in a gym, you need to lift weights that challenge you each time – and it's the same thing here. I do my morning session once I've finished my shower as my wet room becomes particularly steamy and I get a strange satisfaction by blowing the steam out of the window and clearing the room with my breath.

I know this appears to be a lot of work and time consuming, but remember that you can do this anywhere; in the lift, when searching out a place to eat for lunch, while chopping your vegetables for your evening meal. I mean, you're going to be breathing anyway, so why not make it a decent and beneficial activity. Don't worry if you can't do it all from day one. Do what you can and build up to it and remember that anything you do is going to be beneficial.

Soon enough, this type of breathing will become second nature and your regular breathing will also change for the better. And for those of you out there who want six-pack abs; I also noticed that because this uses the stomach a lot, that it also gets a workout. I found that after only a few days my stomach got firmer and more defined. And what's more, for every litre of oxygen consumed, 5 calories are burnt. If that's not reason enough why you should breathe plentiful and deeply, then I don't know what is. You can do that anywhere.

I just want to stress again, particularly if you've not exercised for a while or you're more than just a bit overweight or not used to exercising, you should seek the help of professional personal trainers or instructors. You should also consult your doctor if you have any underlying health issues before you start on any drastic change to your exercising habits. I've seen it too many times where people who have clearly not exercised since school get all keen and join a gym or take up a sport and do too much too soon. They either wind up injured (or worse) and then that puts an end to their exercise routine.

I'm a firm believer in little and often; a slowly *slowly* methodology when it comes to exercise. We've all heard the story of the hare and the tortoise haven't we? Here's an interesting real life example of the hare and tortoise story about a runner called Stu Mittleman. In 1986 Stu entered into a gruelling 1000 mile race (yes, that's not a misprint – one thousand) across the US. While other runners went off and tried to do as much as they could per day, Stu started slowly and ran for several hours less than his fellow competitors. Gradually, over the course of the 11 days, he built up his body to the point where it could cope with running up to 21hrs in a day. He not only won the race, but was also the only person to finish the race too.

Our goal here is to finish the race and not just be super keen and enthusiastic in the beginning. You've heard the expression that good things come to those who wait, well it's true. Be patient with your training and it will pay dividends. That doesn't mean don't push it when the time is right; just go easy at the beginning – especially if you're new to exercise. Speak to a professional about a training regime that will work for you or just introduce the small changes to your daily routine that I've been talking about in this chapter.

Chapter Summary

✓ Exercise plays an imperative role in any healthy lifestyle.
✓ Movement will stimulate the lymph flow and remove toxins from your body.
✓ Undertake whatever exercise you enjoy and aim for 4-6 times a week for around 40 minutes – remember to warm up, warm down and stretch.
✓ Exercise boosts your metabolism.
✓ Three ways to get you up in the morning include asking better questions, getting better sleep and visualisation.
✓ Your cells' first need, and primary food, is oxygen. You learnt a simple breathing technique to help your cells get what they require.

10–Identity and Visualisation

"Imagination is everything" – *Albert Einstein*

"[People] do not attract what they want, but which they are." – *James Allen*

Do you realise that anything you see around you created by humans has been created twice. First it was imagined and created in the mind of someone and then it was created physically. Even the chair that you're probably sitting on was built twice. Albert Einstein come up with the Theory of Relativity and thus changed our understanding of the world because he *imagined* what it would be like to ride on a beam of light. His 'thought experiments' are what gave us these great scientific breakthroughs. The ability to imagine and visualise what we want is perhaps the greatest ability that we possess.

When I moved into my first home, it was a bit of a wreck. A relic from the 1960's which had hardly changed in the 50 years since. I had a vision in my head though about how it would look – even though (as it turned out) it was over a year away from being anything like it is now. As I sit and write this book in that very flat, everything is just as I imagined it those many years before. I first had to create the picture of it in my head *before* it was created in reality. That's what we are going to work on in this chapter - how to create this vision of your perfect 'you' in *your* head, so that you can have it one day in your real life.

Throughout this book I've given you tips and tools on how to make real and lasting changes to help in your weight goals or health and fitness plans. There is one thing that will help move you faster and more assuredly towards that goal - and it is this: how you see yourself. What's your identity as person in relation to health, fitness, weight, size and so on? How you view yourself is the biggest determiner on whether you succeed or not because it's that which will create the standards by which you live and the choices that you will make. And it doesn't matter what you look like now on the outside; what's important is how you see yourself on the inside.

For example if you consider yourself to be someone who is "always battling with your weight" or someone who is "always on a diet", then that's exactly what will be the case. The key here is to get you thinking and really *believing* in a new identity. And I will introduce a few concepts to do that for you and while I do, I want you to remember the exercises on change which were covered earlier and keep an open mind, because some of this might seem a little strange to you at first.

How we talk to ourselves and how we perceive ourselves has a great impact on our lives. If you grew up in a household where you were told by your parents you were no good, or not very pretty or whatever, after a while you start to believe it and act as if it were true. If you believe that you'll always be fat, do you think that you will ever give exercise or a healthy eating plan a proper go? Honestly? I bet not. Because deep down you are expecting it *not* to work and that will re-enforce how you view yourself and also confirm your identity and place in the world. The world will still make sense to you as it always has because your identity in it is intact. If you succeed, however, it's only because you *truly* believe that it's possible for you and because you can identify with the new person - the one you're determined to be - as being you.

I have always held a belief that I'm a fit and active person – even when I sit down and scoff the odd bit of junk food or have not exercised for a while – and because I do, I am always thinking about how the actions I take will affect my identity. Would a fit person do this? How can I make this into some form of exercise? How long do I have to work out to burn this off? Whilst I considered myself to be fit, I didn't necessarily associate myself into being healthy and there is a difference. You can be fit but still be massively unhealthy. I used to exercise for 'damage limitation' and not really be concerned about what I was eating. As I've continued to learn about the body and health, I have become acutely aware that health is really more important than just being fit. As a result, I crafted new questions to incorporate health and ask whether this is something a healthy person would do, and therefore have seen a shift for the better in my food choices.

When you look in the mirror, right into your eyes – who is it you see? Is it someone who is fit, attractive or healthy? Or is it someone who will start some new diet or exercise scheme and give up? Or perhaps is it someone who will battle with the bulge the rest of their life? It could be anything, but I presuppose that it's not something that serves you well if you're reading this book. When you change your identify, you will change your entire approach to what you do, what you eat and everything else.

So the first thing to do is to *decide* on who you want to be. It's a good idea (and fun) to create a new persona. And to do this I've included the following process which I first came across on a course run by an American trainer and UCLA guest lecturer called Joseph McClendon III. It will help to give you focus.

Identity Process

List at least 10 examples for each of the following types of words. They should be words which will inspire you and drive you to succeed in your weight/fitness/health goals. I've listed a couple of examples to get you started.

Adjective (describing words)	Adjective (describing words)	Noun (naming words)	Verb (doing words)
Successful	Adventurous	Athlete	Studies
Confident	Disciplined	Coach	Exercises
Inventive	Flexible	Dad	Trains

Now that you've got the various words, I want you to put a sentence together with three of your favourite and most inspiring words from each column. For example:

"*I, Joe Bloggs, **am a** successful, confident, inventive, disciplined, decisive **and** flexible; coach, athlete **and** dad **that** loves to exercise, trains effortlessly **and** studies health continuously.*"

Play around with it and have fun replacing the words in *italics* with other ones which work for you and leaving the ones in ***bold and italics*** there to give the sentence structure. This is now your 'Morning Power Statement'.

Every morning when you first wake up, have a written copy of your *Morning Power Statement* somewhere close to your mirror. Look yourself in the eyes and say it with conviction and emotion. This is not an affirmation as I don't want you merely repeating this with no passion. It's more of an incantation (like a magical spell or charm). One of the best ways to get e*motion* into something (if you find it challenging) is with *motion*. Move about a bit as you say it to yourself. I know it feels silly, but remember what I said about having an open mind and going for something new and different. Well, this is your chance.

If what you've been trying up to now hasn't worked for you, then you should do something – *anything* else, remember? I've heard it said many times (as I'm sure you have too) that the definition of insanity is doing the same thing over and over and expecting different results (that was Einstein too). Well, now it's time to do something different. I also recommend doing this first thing in the morning, in the first 20 minutes after waking. During this period after waking, your mind is more receptive to information than at other times during the day, so take advantage of that.

Do this for just 30 days and notice what changes happen in your life. If you start to change your identity about health, or exercise, or your weight or anything like that, then everything *around you* will change. As you start to *think* of yourself as someone who is x, y, z (whatever that might be) you will start to *behave* like that. When you're offered that second helping of dessert your unconscious will kick in and you'll be asking yourself "Is this something an x, y, z person would eat/drink/do?" As you have this identity more and more ingrained into you, you'll start to notice these changes. First you must *think* and then you will *be*. Learn to act 'as if'. By that I mean, learn to act *as if* something is already true, even if it's not.

I once heard a story about Donald Trump describing how he started out. The story goes that he went round to several banks and investors in New York looking to secure capital for a development he wanted to start. He kept introducing himself as a property developer – despite the fact he'd never done any property developing up to that point! Despite that one small challenge, he did secure millions of dollars in funding simply by acting '*as if*'. By acting '*as if*', that vision of being a property developer became 'so' for him. Even when he lost all his money in the early 90's and used to joke that even the homeless person in the street was richer then he was (he was *billions* of dollars in debt), he still *saw* himself as a successful and wealthy person and so wasn't broke for very long. So act '*as if*' you are a top class athlete, act '*as if*' you are someone who can walk that bit further each day, act '*as if*' you are someone who puts health above all else – whatever it might be for you.

Another way to help this process along is, as I've mentioned before, to have more awareness and consciousness about what you're doing. So if you accept that extra doughnut, do it consciously and think through the consequences. Take time to stop and ask yourself questions about that action?

> *"Is this moving me towards or away from my goals of ....?"*

> *"What will it cost me if I eat/do this......?"*

> *"How can I still be included in the group and stay healthy?"*

> *"How much exercise will I need to do to burn this off?"*

These are just examples and I suggest to you that you come up with a list of your own questions which you can ask yourself at times when your resolve is tested. Initially, asking yourself these questions will be a bit time consuming and alien to you, but after a while it will become second nature. You're already doing that process - just with different questions and extremely rapidly. *"Mmm, I wonder what this tastes like?", "that looks nice, doesn't it?"* and so on. This will become the same after a while if you start to do it consciously often enough and after a while it will become unconscious and quick.

Another thing to look at when changing your identity is to reflect on your environment. Is it the environment that an 'X' person would be in (substitute 'X' for the kind of person you want to be)? What about the company you keep? Do you have friends that you only see down the pub and over a few drinks? Is it time to start taking a look at your surroundings and the people you hang out with and determine whether it fits in with the new you? It might be hard to accept, but there may (in all likelihood, will) have to be some drastic changes. Do you always go on that Starbucks run with the gang or head out for that Friday fry-up? I know; it's a way of socialising and building and maintaining relationships but let's not forget the most important relationship here – the one with yourself. If that's gone then what use are the others? Let's evaluate some of this right now.

On the lines below, identify all the times in the week, (or the activities) that do not really line up with the identity that you have created for yourself.

_____
_____
_____
_____
_____
_____
_____
_____
_____
_____
_____
_____
_____
_____
_____
_____
_____
_____
_____
_____
_____
_____
_____

Now, for each of those activities, write down what it is that you are getting from them, for example: friendship, possible promotion, escapism, peace, interesting conversation...

_____

_____

_____

_____

_____

_____

_____

_____

_____

_____

_____

_____

_____

_____

_____

_____

_____

_____

_____

_____

_____

_____

_____

_____

_____

_____

_____

_____

_____

_____

_____

_____

_____

Now write down some alternatives, which would fit into your new identity, and be good choices which also satisfy the need you identified. For example, if you presently go to the pub to maintain a friendship, could you maintain that friendship by having that person over for dinner instead, or taking up golf or squash, or maybe something else? I believe that there's always an alternative, you just have to ask yourselves the question *how? How* can I still satisfy 'X' *and* still be healthy in the process? Or *how* can I still maintain my relationship with 'X' *and* be true to my new identity?

Come up with your own *'how'* question below for each of your activities and then your unconscious will seek out the answers. Write the alternatives down below too.

How _____?

Alternatives

_____

_____

_____

_____

_____

_____

How _____?

Alternatives

_____

_____

_____

_____

_____

_____

How _____?

Alternatives

_____

_____

_____

_____

_____

_____

How _____?

Alternatives

_____

_____

_____

_____

_____

_____

How _____?

Alternatives

_____

_____

_____

_____

_____

_____

The other thing that is crucially important when changing your identity is to really *see* yourself as that new you. When you look in the mirror, it's important to see the person you *will* become and not the person you might be at that present time. I encourage you to get pictures, either from magazines, the internet, or your past with the body of how you want to be. Put a picture of your own head onto those pictures or obscure the face in some way. It's important that you associate yourself into that image rather than idolise another person. Have the images somewhere where you will see them often. When you look at that image, take a minute or two to really get into the feeling of that image.

➤ *How do you feel now that you are _____?*

➤ *What are others saying about you now that you've achieved _____?*

➤ *What can you do now that you couldn't before because of this change?*

➤ *What can you wear now?*

➤ *Where can you go?*

Really get into the feelings and lifestyle of the future you. When visualising your future you, it's also really important to visualise your future 'you' carrying out the steps required to get to that point. Otherwise you might just get stuck in a fantasy of how you want to be but not see yourself taking the necessary steps. Picture yourself eating and exercising correctly with enjoyment and ease – not just that finale scene. You need to be able to associate your identity with someone who takes action and does the work to get the job done. Not just have it handed to you.

Place any pictures which will help you with visualising the process and the outcome in areas where you might have previously gone for a snack. Perhaps stick it to the inside of your cupboard, with questions or phrases perhaps underneath to encourage you to stick to your plan of healthy eating and exercise.

It's important to immerse yourself with as much positive and goal focussed imagery as you can, as this will penetrate into your unconscious mind and then it will be what you end up focussing on. What you focus on is what you tend to get. You need to make sure that you focus on what you want by surrounding yourself with positive images and thus ensure that your mind is aligned to your goal. Have you ever bought something new: a new car, handbag, dress or jacket and then noticed that it's suddenly everywhere? This is because you tend to only notice and pay attention to things you focus on. There are 4 billion bits of information around us at any one time. The mind takes in 2000 bits of that 4 billion but only consciously processes about 3 bits (previously it was thought the brain processed 7 ± 2 bits but recent research suggests it's as little as 3)! So you have to delete out a lot of the information around you.

We do *become* what we *think* about *most* of the time. So think the right things and you will notice the changes. In the 1960's, when plastic surgery was taking off, the famous American plastic surgeon and author of the book Psycho-Cybernetics, Maxwell Maltz, noticed that although the physical appearance of a person might have changed, psychologically they still had a poor self image. The patients were first attempting to change their *external* environment before working on their *internal* environment and so the superficial results they achieved on the outside did not make them feel any happier.

Maltz sought to find a way of assisting these patients and helped them set the goal of a positive outcome by *visualising* that positive outcome. It seemed to work and he was fascinated why setting goals should give these results. He discovered that by having a self-affirmation and using mental visualisation techniques it created a powerful connection between the mind and the body. Maltz specified techniques in which people needed to create positive inner goals as the means by which they could develop positive outer goals. The focus on altering inner attitudes first and visualising the goal as the person wants it, is paramount to his approach, as a person's outer success can never be more than the one visualized internally.

We must program our minds to take in the information and the instructions that will benefit us. It's the classic 'garbage in - garbage out' result. How can you hope to feel great if all you do is ask yourself "why am I so fat?", "why am I overweight?", or "why can't I fit into this outfit?" Start by putting the right kind of programming into your mind. Think of your mind much like a computer. It can perform all manner of tasks and activities for you but it needs the right software and programming in order to do it. Install faulty software and your computer will start to malfunction. Know that you are the programmer to the software which runs *your* computer and make sure that you program that software in a way that serves you right.

Chapter Summary

✓ Visualisation is the key to accomplishing many of your goals. You must see it in your mind before you see it in reality.

✓ Visualise yourself as you *want* to be and not how you are *currently*.

✓ You started to work on asking yourself better questions about how you can make this change in your life.

✓ You came up with a new and improved identity for yourself – your Morning Power Statement.

11 - Goals

Now that we're almost at the end of our journey together, let's discuss goals. The importance of setting goals has been spoken about so much that, if you're like me, you probably take it all a bit for granted. "Yeah, I know all about goal setting", "yeah, they have to be SMART – specific, measurable, achievable, realistic and time-bound. Yeah, I know all this." Well, do you actually do any of this? Do you write your goals down and review them regularly? The challenge is that because we hear it so much, we tend to just ignore it. So just to make sure that you leave my company with the best possible chance of success I'm going to introduce you to the method I follow for goal setting. I've brought together the best bits from methods I've come across and call it 'The Kaly Method' (Kaly means good in Greek!) and it involves 13 steps.

The Kaly Method

1. **Decide**: The first step with any goal is to decide what it is you *really* want? Make sure that it's something that *you've* decided and not what you think someone *else* wants for you. It doesn't

matter what it is as long as it's something that you have a level of control over. So instead of saying that your goal is for 'so and so' to notice your hot body, say that your goal is to be an example of health and vitality (and this will naturally attract the right people to you anyway). Decide on *what* you want *before* you decide on whether or not it's *possible*. Right now, it's just about what it is and not how you're going to achieve it. Remember that the goal must be about you and not others.

2. **Why**: Determine *why* you want the goal in the first place. If you have a big enough why, you'll figure out the how. Make it exciting and something worth striving for. A goal like "I want to lose loads of weight" isn't going to inspire you as much as a goal such as "I want to look and feel smoking hot for my trip to Miami". By now, you should already have many compelling reasons *why* you want to achieve your goal from our work together earlier.

3. **Faith**: You might be unsure on how you will achieve your goal but you must have faith, an absolute belief that it is possible. Have unrealistic expectations of success. The thing is that in order for you to even *conceive* of a goal, somewhere inside of you, you must have some idea for how it's going to be achieved. You might not know it right now and that's okay. Using some of the techniques in this book will help you to instil belief changes. For example the visualisation exercises, the Swish Pattern and the belief change process will all help.

4. **Deadlines**: There are no unrealistic goals, just unrealistic deadlines. Every goal should have a deadline. Otherwise it's just a dream. But what

happens if you miss the deadline? You set another one, of course. Just because you missed your target of 66kg by June 1st doesn't mean that you give up; re-focus and you might hit it by September. And if you miss that? Guess what? You set another and another until you get what you want. Remember, if you have a big enough why then the goal is worth the time and effort.

5. **Penmanship**: Commit that goal to paper. When you write it down, make it detailed and specific. We've already discussed the fact that your unconscious mind takes everything at face value and will throw back to you generalities if you give it generalities. There's an often cited 'Yale Goal Study' which states that in 1953 a group of researchers interviewed graduating seniors about their goals and found only 3% had any clear written goals. When the researchers reassessed the graduates twenty years on in 1973, the 3% who had written goals had a personal wealth more than that of the other 97% combined! I've not actually been able to validate whether this study is actually true or not, but from my own experience, I know that writing down goals makes them more achievable. It seems as though there is a strange connection between writing a goal down and it being planted in your unconscious -automatically making it that much more achievable. In addition, when writing goals, follow the *3P Penmanship* approach – make it Personal, in the Present tense and Positive. By that I mean use "I......" in your statement. The goal should be written as if you have already achieved it and it be stated in the positive. Here are a couple of examples.

BAD Example:

"I want to lose 3 kilos by next year."

GOOD Example

"I weigh 75kgs and feel happier and healthier than ever before!"

Although the first example uses the first 'P' (personal), it omits the next two. It's projecting into the future by saying 'next year' (I've never seen a calendar with the word 'tomorrow' written on it!) and the goal is a negative goal talking about how much that person wants to 'lose'.

The goal should also include the date that you see yourself having achieved it and contain emotionally inspiring words in order to get you excited about achieving the goal.
For example:

"It's the first of May 2014 and I'm walking down the beach in Thailand feeling so healthy, relaxed and energised with the sun beating down on my back. I weigh between 72 and 74 kg's and feel absolutely fantastic. And better still, I now know exactly how easy and effortless it is to maintain my ideal weight range and my confidence levels are sky high!"

Write your goal here or in your notebook:

_____

_____

_____

_____

_____

_____

_____

_____

_____

_____

6. **Present**: Where are you right now? What's your health like? How much do you weigh? What is your fitness level currently? Would you set off on a road trip without knowing where it was you were starting from? Even with having the best map in the world and knowing the destination, it would still be a struggle if you didn't know where you were to start with – even the GPS navigation system in your car spends a few minutes working out where it is, doesn't it? Spend some time now to write down where it is you are presently on the route to achieving your goal.

_____

_____

_____

_____

_____

_____

_____

_____

_____

_____

_____

_____

_____

_____

_____

_____

7. **Challenges**: As soon as you set a goal, you'll start to come up against obstacles and challenges determined to thwart you. It's better to figure these out now so you're better prepared for them when they rear their ugly heads. Do you have a sweet tooth? A desire for junk food? Too many people urging you out to the pub at lunch time?

_____

_____

_____

_____

_____

_____

_____

_____

_____

_____

_____

_____

_____

_____

_____

_____

_____

8. **Ability**: What abilities will you need in order to achieve your goal? What skills and knowledge? Do you already have some level of knowledge? Most probably you will need to acquire more skills and knowledge so work out what these are and how you can get them. Luckily, you already have some essential skills, knowledge and key tips and facts by having read this book, so you're already well on the way to success! Use the space below to include all the skills you might need.

_____

_____

_____

_____

_____

_____

_____

_____

_____

_____

_____

_____

_____

_____

_____

_____

_____

9. **Connection**: No one achieves anything on their own. There are no _self_-made millionaires – despite what you might think. Even they need customers don't they? To be a top Olympian you need a coach, but even if what you strive for is just a healthier you, chances are that you'll get there quicker connecting with people and getting their help. You might need a personal trainer, the support of your family or maybe even the advice in this book! Write down who it is that you need to connect with and enlist to help you achieve your goal.

_____

_____

_____

_____

_____

_____

_____

_____

_____

10. **Plan**: If it's not written down then it's not getting done. Would you trust someone to build you an extension on your house without seeing the written plan and technical drawings? A plan will give you structure and guidance and something to measure against. As Peter Drucker, the well respected and influential management consultant says: "What gets measured gets managed." Write down all the things that you need to do, and then what order and priority these need to be in. It doesn't have to be perfect. As General George S Patten said: "A good plan violently executed today is far and away better than a perfect plan tomorrow." Write a list of things you need to do below.

_____

_____

_____

_____

_____

_____

_____

_____

_____

_____

_____

_____

_____

_____

_____

_____

_____

_____

_____

_____

11. **Momentum**: Do something towards your goal every single day. It might just be reading your goal, maybe making a phone call or sending an email. Isaac Newton, the famous scientist, told us that momentum pushes us forward and it's a lot easier to keep something moving than to start moving it from a stationary position. This is as true for your goals as it is for anything else. Use the law of momentum to get you there.

12. **Morning Visualisation**: We examined just how important it is to be able to visualise yourself in achievement of the goal. Create some imagery of how you see that goal manifesting and focus on it every day. Remember that it's equally important to visualise the process as well as the outcome so that you actually do the steps necessary to get the outcome. Read your written goal aloud each morning and get excited by it. Here's a visualisation technique that I first learnt from Joseph McClendon III that I use and you might want to as well.

   a. First thing when you wake up, read your goal aloud repeatedly while listening to some inspiring music. Move around, dance, rebound -whatever it is to get the juices flowing.

   b. Spend about a song doing that, reading the goal aloud over and over.

c.   When the second uplifting track comes on, start to picture in your mind having achieved that goal. Use printed pictures from magazines or the internet if you find it helps.

d.   Have a written statement – a 'future pace statement' - describing what it's like 6 to 12 months after having achieved your goal. Let's say your goal was to be able to run round your local park by January. Your future pace statement might be something like seeing yourself in July running in a 10k race.

Here's some space to write down your 'future pace statement'.

_____

_____

_____

_____

_____

_____

_____

_____

_____

_____

e.   Read your 'future pace statement' during the third track once and while stationary.

f.   Then see out the rest of the music track (while restarting to jump around, dance whatever) by visualising that 'future pace' 6/12 months after the attainment of the original goal (no need for actual picture on this one).

13.   **Evening Visualisation**: At the end of each day, re-read your goal aloud (not your 'future pace') just

before turning in for bed, so that your unconscious mind can go to work on it overnight for you.

So that's it - The Kaly Method to goal setting. By following this and the rest of the advice in the book, you are now in a great position to start making *lasting* changes in your life.

Chapter Summary

✓ Only 3% of people have written goals.
✓ Writing your goals down will make them more achievable.
✓ Use The Kaly Method to goal setting to structure your goals.

---

12 – A Final Word

"Take the first step in faith. You don't have to see the whole staircase, just take the first step." - Martin Luther King, Jr

"Once we're thrown off our habitual paths, we think all is lost, but it's only here that the new and the good begins." - Leo Tolstoy

Well done for coming with me on this journey! You've kept me company and completed this book – this is evidence that you're prepared to put the work in to make this area of your life a success. So many people say they want change and then buy a book or sign up to a program and never finish it, so the fact that you've made it, completed the exercises and are here with me means that you're a winner already and taking the next steps will be easy.

I hope that you have worked through this book in the way it was intended and have taken advantage of all it has to offer. The truth of the matter is; that to become fit, healthy and happy does take work. There are no real shortcuts to anything worthwhile in life, but it can be an exciting and rewarding journey. By reviewing your beliefs and values and having the skills and abilities to change them, this alone will set you off in the right direction. You have taken the first step by reading this book and because you are now armed with this knowledge, you're in a better position than ever before to succeed. Now that you have already started to make these small changes to your life, you'll realise that it is simple and it will appear as though it doesn't take much effort at all.

Now that you have read the book through once, go back and *re*-view what you have learnt. What are the differences for you that are already making the difference? Again, I want to thank you for allowing me to be here to guide you on your way and I very much appreciate all the effort that you have already put in. I would love to hear about your experiences with this book and for you to tell me your success stories. Please send me your 'before and after' photos or any personal tales to info@thethoughtgym.com and perhaps they can get included in subsequent editions.

I hope that you realise now that we all have it in our power to choose how we behave and that by working-out the mind first, you'll get what you want elsewhere. It's been a great experience for me to be able share with you all this information and I hope that you will now join me in believing that *"if you train the mind...the body will follow*™*"*.

To your ongoing health, wealth and happiness!

Hari

"You may never know what results come from your action. But if you do nothing, there will be no result." - Gandhi

"All that we are is the result of what we have thought. The mind is everything. What we think we become." - Buddha

Further Information

I have taken what I have learnt and given it to you to use with the intention of helping you to make positive changes in your life. My advice comes from both my life experiences and learning from others. Everything in this book I have personally done, or still do and whilst this book is written from my own findings and experiences, I have been fortunate enough to learn from a great many other sources. I can recommend the following list as good places to start for increasing your understanding on some of the concepts discussed in this book and also further reading.

1. Tony Robbins (2001), *'Unlimited Power'*, Pocket Books, ISBN 978-0743409391
2. Richard Bandler & John Grinder (1989), *'The Structure of Magic'*, Science and Behavior Books, ISBN 978-0831400446
3. John Grinder and Carmen Bostic-St Clair (2001), *'Whispering in the Wind'*, J & C Enterprises, ISBN 978-0971722309
4. Richard Bandler & John Grinder (1990), *'Frogs into Princes: Introduction to Neurolinguistic*

Programming', Eden Grove Editions, ISBN 978-1870845038

5. Joseph O'Conner & John Seymour (2003), *'Introducing NLP'*, Thorsons, ISBN 978-1855383449

6. Richard Wiseman (2009), *'59 Seconds: Think a little, change a lot'*, Macmillan, ISBN 978-0-230-74429-5

7. Sue Knight (2009), *'NLP at Work'*, Nicholas Brealey Publishing, ISBN 978-1857885293

8. Joseph O'Conner and Andrea Lages (2004), *'Coaching with NLP'*, Element ISBN 978-0007151226

9. David Molden and Pat Hutchinson (2010), *'Brilliant NLP Workbook'*, Prentice Hall Business, ISBN 978-0273737438

10. John Robbins (1998), *'Diet for a New America'*, H J Kramer, ISBN 978-0915811816

11. John Robbins (2010), *'The Food Revolution'*, Conari Press, ISBN 978-1573244879

12. Allen Carr (2010), *'Lose Weight Now'*, Arcturus Publishing Ltd, ISBN 978-1848377202

13. Paul McKenna (2007), *'I Can Make You Thin'*, Bantam Press, ISBN 978-0593060926

14. Jorge Cruise (2003), *'8 Minutes in the Morning'*, Rodale International Ltd, ISBN 978-1405021012

15. Lloyd Bradley (2009), *'The Rough Guide to Men's Health'*, Rough Guides, ISBN 978-1848360044

16. Matt Roberts (2011), *'Fitness For Life Manual'*, Dorling Kindersley, ISBN 978-1405392426

17. Dr John Briffa (1999), *'Bodywise'*, CICO Books, ISBN 978-1903116012

18. Dr Robert Young (2009), *'The pH Miracle'*, Piatkus, ISBN 978-0749939816

19. Colin Campbell (2006), *'The China Study'*, Ben Bella, ISBN 978-1932100662

20. Brian Tracy (2010), *'Goals'*, Berrett-Koehler, ISBN 978-1605094113

21. Tony Robbins, *'Living Health'*, Audio CD Training, tonyrobbins.com

22. Tony Robbins , *'The Body You Deserve'*, Audio CD Training, tonyrobbins.com

23. Joseph McClendon III (2011), *'The Next Step Seminar'*, josephmcclendon.net

24. Further audio courses from: Tony Robbins, Bob Proctor, Brian Tracy, Zig Ziglar, Les Brown, Deepak Chopra

25. Courses in hypnotherapy and NLP by Toby & Kate McCartney tobyandkatemccartney.com

Keep in touch with me via...

 thethoughtgym.com

 facebook.com/thethoughtgym

 twitter.com/thethoughtgym

 youtube.com/thethoughtgym

About the author

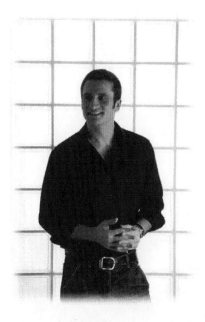

Hari Kalymnios studied Physics with Astrophysics at the University of Manchester where he earned a First Class Honours degree. Following his degree, Hari's continued desire to learn and grow saw him spend three years independently travelling the world, meeting and getting to know a variety of people and cultures. On returning to the UK, Hari settled into a city profession, however his real passion lay in health and fitness which led him to pursue those areas instead. Frustrated at seeing colleagues feeling lacklustre, de-energised or suffering with their health or weight, Hari sought to understand what it was that made the difference. Why is it that some people can be the size they want, exercise (or accomplish whatever their goals in life are) when others can't? Hari wanted to know the reason. His research led him to studying several fields including health, fitness, nutrition, psychology and NLP amongst others. Distilling the most useful parts of his research, coupled with his own lifetime of experiences, Hari has detailed in an extremely easy-to-read and companion-led book, the steps needed for a person to make noticeable shifts in their thinking. And hence be able to take perceptible and genuine steps to achieving their goals.

Hari is 35 years old and lives in London where he runs his website and business for helping people achieve their health goals – www.TheThoughtGym.com